It's Really Rather Normal

Tilly Gerritsma and Titus Rivas

It's Really Rather Normal:
A different view on hearing voices and seeing images

Tilly Gerritsma & Titus Rivas, MA

Lulu.com

Dedicated to my sons

In memory of the overly controversial Dutch parapsychologist W.H.C. Tenhaeff

Development is evolution, evolution is transcendence
Ken Wilber, *The Atman Project.*

I now consider it possible that each of us is a continuing spiritual essence lasting over time, and occasionally incarnated in a human body.
Carl Rogers, *Speaking Personally*

It's Really Rather Normal is a translation of the book *Gek Genoeg Gewoon*, originally published by Ankh-Hermes, Deventer, The Netherlands, in 2007 (ISBN: 9789020284645).

Lulu.com, 2013. ISBN 978-1-291-50857-4

Contents

Acknowledgments

We are grateful to Chris Canter, Dr. Sandra Escher, Ron Coleman, and Paul Baker for their constructive comments and references. Also, we owe thanks to Mrs. Anny Dirven for her assistance while we were writing this book and to Mrs. Elisabeth Hallett for proofreading the manuscript.

Introduction by Titus Rivas

Near the end of 2005, I was approached, much to my surprise, by Tilly Gerritsma of Mill, a seasoned experiential expert in the field of hearing voices and related subjects.

Evidently, she had read some of my work and believed I could be a suitable co-author for a book she had wanted to write for some time. After several meetings at my home in Nijmegen, various phone calls, and numerous e-mails, I concluded that the project would be interesting enough for me to want to take part in it. My particular task would consist of formulating a few structuring questions, critically reading over Tilly's text, and presenting a brief overview of insights taken from the literature about these subjects.

My own relevant background is rather diverse.

First of all, I have acquired, if I may say so, quite a broad expertise in the fields of parapsychology and psychical research. Among other things, I published a general written course about this topic, a concise encyclopedic book, and several specialist works about research into reincarnation and survival after death, besides numerous articles, reviews, and columns. I have also carried out numerous field studies in psychical research, which means that I have tried to reconstruct and evaluate the spontaneous experiences of a varied sample of subjects.

In general, parapsychology or psychical research deals with paranormal experiences, in other words with experiences that do not seem to fit into the mainstream scientific or materialist world view. In parapsychology, we are usually open to the possibility that such experiences cannot always be reduced to hallucinations or delusions, and that they can sometimes be linked to an objective or inter-subjective reality that also exists separately from the person in question. At least, this is the kind of parapsychology of which I am a proponent. I do not feel any affinity with a skeptical type of parapsychology, represented by scholars such as Richard Wiseman, Christopher French, or Susan Blackmore, who are trying to reduce all paranormal experiences to psychological or even physiological processes. I obviously endorse the principle of skeptics such as the late Dutch philosopher Joop Doorman, that we ought to show respect for ideological differences, but I am struck by the fact that, particularly among skeptics, there is, in practice, very little room for such respect.

Apart from the foregoing, it seems relevant to note that I have Master's degrees in both theoretical psychology and systematic philosophy. My studies in theoretical psychology have given me enough general knowledge of the subject, so that I am aware of theoretical concepts such as Freud's unconscious, the non-conscious processes of cognitivism, the Jungian subconscious, etc.

During my psychology studies, I already met several psychiatric patients through my fellow students. I noticed how different all these people were, despite the very limited number of psychiatric labels applied to them. Furthermore, it was precisely in this period (mid to late nineties) that the acceptance of organic factors in psychiatric syndromes evidently led to a very one-sided treatment of patients. Although there were talks with social psychiatric nurses that seemed to be of little importance, there was a strong emphasis on medication.

More concretely, the personal fate of a friend of mine prompted me to read widely about the current theories concerning schizophrenia. I found it remarkable that the Nijmegen RIAGG (Regional Institute for Ambulatory Mental Health Care) that took care of him seemed to be completely convinced of the value of the bio-psychiatric approach to this construct of schizophrenia. According to this approach it was no longer necessary to look for emotional, psycho-dynamic, or existential factors, i.e., for specifically psychological problems. I felt this was quite strange because psychological problems are present in the lives of anyone outside psychiatry; it did not seem reasonable to assume they would suddenly stop being of importance in the lives of psychiatric patients.

Even if there are important organic factors in schizophrenia (assuming that this construct really matches a clearly demarcated part of reality), this still does not mean that the person in question can suddenly be reduced to a soulless robot. I did find that this point was being recognized to a certain extent among adherents of cognitive approaches to schizophrenia, which – in contrast to the one-sided biological approach – stressed the importance of irreducible psychological factors, such as one's own beliefs about schizophrenia. Within the RIAGG itself, they were mainly talking about the acceptance of the syndrome and the limitations that were, in their view, inevitably and permanently linked to schizophrenia or to the side-effects of medication.

Moreover, I now know there are serious investigators, such as the Dutch psychiatrist Marius Romme, who deny the scientific value of the construct of schizophrenia, something which, during my studies, I only read about in the context of anti-psychiatry. Their findings show that the concept of schizophrenia is not at all based on good research, and that it lacks all scientific validity. It essentially amounts to a pseudo-scientific conventional concept that is used at the expense of the well-being and vitality of psychiatric patients. Psychiatrists are also searching for neurological factors (with or without a genetic component) because of the 'medical' approach implied by the construct of schizophrenia and they tend to ignore any psychological context or meaning of the symptoms, thereby alienating the patient from his or her own life. This makes the experiences of people around me all the more shocking.

Unfortunately, someone in my personal environment took his own life. A friend in my neighborhood had been suicidal for a very long time when, after 16 years, he finally succeeded in taking his life in 1996. Especially during the last years before his death, he and his friends and acquaintances repeatedly tried to alert psychiatric professionals, but it turned out these had simply labeled him 'incurable'. He was supposed to be a *borderline* patient and this diagnosis made any search for underlying motives of his general attitude seem futile.

On the other hand, my studies in philosophy made me aware how little we really know about the world we live in. For instance, from a rational point of view, it cannot be ruled out a priori that we are actually sharing some kind of *collective dream*, a purely mental reality that exclusively consists of dream images. This 'exotic' possibility is known as ontological idealism and it has been supported by prominent philosophers. In a sense, it is often the foundation of Eastern philosophies. According to Hinduism, Buddhism, Jainism and Sikhism, we could ultimately reach a state of enlightenment by getting rid of our illusions about reality. This awareness of the relative uncertainty of the basic nature of reality has motivated me to be as explicit as possible about my own positions. For example, I still believe that apart from our inner lives there is also a shared physical world, and that there is an interaction between ourselves as psychological beings, our bodies, material objects, and other beings with an inner life.

Nonetheless, I believe the prevalent scientific ontology (world view), materialism, is less plausible than the idealism I have just mentioned. This is because you can intellectually 'delete' the objective existence of a physical, external reality from your world view, but you certainly cannot do this with your own inner world of subjectivity. If our inner world is merely an illusion, meaning that it would not really exist, then any reason to believe in an outer world immediately disappears. The physical world can only be known *through* our inner world, via our consciousness. This is a position known as Neo-Cartesianism, because, just as René Descartes did, it acknowledges the epistemic primacy of one's own consciousness over the possible (though, for many, still plausible) existence of a material reality.

This implies we need to be respectful toward anybody's subjective experience. We cannot get to know physical reality directly, but only via our consciousness, and therefore it is indefensible to interpret anyone's subjective experience as delusional as soon as it does not agree with what others believe they know about the world inter-subjectively.

This does not mean, by the way, that there are no standards anymore to make a well-founded distinction between things that only exist within someone's personal subjective experience and things that are part of the inter-subjective experience of a shared reality. Within my own conception of things there certainly are *real* 'hallucinations' with no direct link to reality outside the mind and *real* 'delusions', by which I here mean: perceptions or beliefs that really do not match the external world. Thus, somebody may suffer from a delusion that he is in fact not a human being, but an alien who landed on earth only fairly recently. It may be difficult to prove conclusively that this belief is wrong, but we can show that it is very probable that the belief is delusional, precisely because the delusion does not only concern the person's own inner world, but also relates to verifiable external or inter-subjective facts. Similarly, someone may have a hallucination that he is in direct communion with God and that God orders him to massacre a whole village of Native Americans. In this case it seems even more plausible that such a person has lost touch with outer reality, because at any rate the Christian God would never give such an order; on a purely logical level it simply does not match the loving nature of such a divinity.

For these reasons, it remains sensible also for me to recognize that some people may really have certain psychiatric problems. The point is that I would look at psychological reasons for such problems as well and not only at possible neurological causes. There are also cases in which I reject any kind of psychiatric approach, simply because I do not believe there really is a psychiatric disorder involved, but only neutral psychological processes or even totally 'sane' so-called paranormal experiences (in the sense of parapsychology or psychical research). In this respect, I completely agree with Tilly Gerritsma.

Regarding this English version: it is a free translation of the original Dutch text. Readers are welcome to alert us to any errors they may encounter, both in vocabulary and grammar.

I think this is enough as a general introduction.

Titus Rivas

You can buy the book via: http://www.lulu.com/spotlight/itsnormal

Experiences with images and sounds that lack a direct sensory source

by Titus Rivas M.Sc., M.A.

In her dissertation, Sandra Escher refers to a definition of hallucinations, which she derives from Slade and Bentall. A hallucination is any experience that seems to be perceptual and (a) takes place in the absence of an adequate stimulus, (b) has the power or impact of the corresponding (real) perceptual experience, and (c) cannot be directly and voluntarily controlled by the experient.

Hallucinations can be distinguished from (perceptual) *illusions*. These are inadequate interpretations of sensory impressions, which means that relevant stimuli are not physically absent.

Greek philosopher Aristotle already realized that there is a completely natural parallel to hallucinations in our night life, namely in our dreams and nightmares. In these nightly episodes, visual and auditive experiences may occur that are not directly based on sensory impressions. In general, nobody is surprised by such experiences. Only their specific form may surprise us.

Daydreaming or the visualization of situations (for example during meditation) accompanied by vivid images, sounds and odors, is an accepted, normal phenomenon. The mental imagination of images and sounds is an indispensable part of conscious fantasies, but also of creative processes like composing a piece of music or writing a novel. This phenomenon is frequently apparent when we are reading stories as well. Imagination plays an important part within human cognition.

It is very different when these impressions manifest spontaneously and involuntarily during the day, while you're experiencing a waking state of consciousness. Under such circumstances, sounds and images may often seem strange to the person experiencing them. It may seem as if the person in

13

question is dreaming while being awake. Many people associate this with mild psychiatric symptoms or even with a so-called psychosis, a very confused state of mind in which one loses touch with reality.

Thanks to the work of, among others, Dutch researchers Marius Romme and Sandra Escher, we now know this is misguided. Spontaneously seeing all kinds of images or hearing voices and other sounds also happens to individuals without psychiatric problems, who mostly will not be bothered by them and who are able to handle this phenomenon well. The so-called Nemesis-study carried out by the Dutch Trimbos Institute demonstrated that about 17.5% of the normal population had experienced one or more 'psychotic experiences', such as hearing voices, seeing things, or undergoing delusions.

We can already deduce from dreams or visualizations, but also from lively memories, that subjective impressions often are only indirectly related to sensory stimuli, and the study I just mentioned demonstrates that sounds and images may also enter our consciousness involuntarily while, psychiatrically speaking, nothing is wrong.

This means that there is no general relationship between hearing voices or seeing 'visionary' images and a psychiatric disorder. These kinds of phenomena are first of all *neutral* expressions of human possibilities. Only on the basis of someone's general functioning can we determine whether they are connected to psychiatric problems or not.

Undergoing impressions without a direct sensory counterpart is as a neutral phenomenon, a neutral variation of human nature, and it depends on the context in which it occurs and the way the person in question is dealing with it, where it will lead in specific cases.

From a purely logical viewpoint, unconnected to any specific psychiatric theoretical tradition, we can make all kinds of distinctions between different kinds of sounds and images that do not have a direct sensory source. We may classify the experiences, based on the different modalities that are used, in auditory, visual, olfactory or tactile experiences, and so on. While undergoing these impressions, the persons in question may realize that, as such, the images or sounds only exist in their own minds, or rather believe that they reach them directly from the physical world outside.

Furthermore, we can make distinctions based on the supposed source of the experiences. In theory, they may derive from unconscious or subconscious processes within the person himself, but also from external sources, such as telepathy with other people, or contact with spirits of the deceased, or higher beings. For some, such as Tilly Gerritsma, this distinction cannot be drawn very sharply, because in their view all psychical or subjective beings would form a spiritual unity on a deeper level.

Another distinction can be made between, on the one hand, voices and other experiences that the person who undergoes them finds hard to deal with, because they seem to be domineering or disturb one's inner peace, and on the other hand, experiences that do not cause any trouble, or even lead to insight, growth, and joy.

Yet another common distinction we may acknowledge, is the one between experiences that match physical reality and experiences that clearly contain incorrect information. In the first case, it is possible that we are dealing with memories that are forgotten and irretrievable, but also with so-called paranormal or extra-sensory information, such as can be found in (real) clairvoyant or telepathic impressions.
In theory, paranormal information may be the result of subconscious paranormal talents of the person in question, but it may also derive from higher or lower spiritual beings.

In fact, these are the same possibilities that we already know from the realm of dreaming. Dreams may contain paranormal information, but more often than not, they simply build around memories of normal sensory impressions and around fantasies. There are also bizarre dreams or nightmares about demons, and spiritual dreams about a spiritual world in which one can connect with more elevated beings. They can be a source of positive feelings, but they may also lead to anxiety.

A psychiatry that would endorse a humane approach would not primarily focus upon the dichotomy between *normal* versus *abnormal*, but on the way people themselves experience and interpret their own functioning. Such a psychiatry would have to look exclusively at the extent to which someone becomes confused because of his or her voices or visions, is troubled by them, or becomes alienated from the environment.

When someone is no longer able to distinguish between such inner experiences and the outside world, deals with them in an uncritical way, or becomes angry or aggressive, we are clearly facing a psychological or psychiatric problem. This means that people cannot function well in everyday life anymore, because of symptoms such as a lack of concentration at work or sleeplessness. Persons who are suffering from this problem may seem distracted or absent, but also suspicious because their voices tell them that their conversational partner is lying to them. Also, they may laugh at jokes the voices are making, or get angry about certain remarks, or afraid they will be punished if they do not do certain things. People who hear voices and are troubled by their hallucinations may seem tired and so caught up in fear that they shut out others and seem devoid of emotion. Their voices may manifest in a negative way because they are prohibiting things or judging or condemning the person hearing them for certain acts or feelings. Such a negative judgment or condemnation may be accompanied by a form of punishment or even self-mutilation.

Although we need more research, it seems that people who really are affected negatively by hearing voices, are characterized more often by:

- doubting one's own abilities, fear of failure, and insecurity;
- being less positive about oneself;
- being very demanding toward oneself or others, perfectionism;
- attaching a lot of importance to the opinion of others for a basic feeling of self-esteem;
- frustration or disillusionment about oneself or about life, feelings of impotence;

- experiencing one or more traumatic events in life

Thus, it is not the voices or images themselves that are at issue, but rather the way in which these are interpreted and the extent to which the person remains in charge of his or her own life.

The main difference between 'patients' and 'non-patients' seems to be that the latter have more control over their lives and don't feel incapacitated, and also that they hear positive voices more often and have a more positive attitude toward life. Another difference found in studies is that they are not afraid of their voices. They also have more friends and more contacts than patients. It is not necessary that the voices disappear, but it is essential that people are capable of dealing with them positively.

Where do voices and images come from?
Let us now take a brief look at various models and approaches to the question of how hallucinations originate. For this, I have made use of sources such as a brochure of *Stichting Weerklank* (Foundation Resonance), and the works of Marius Romme and Sandra Escher of the section of Social Psychiatry at the University of Maastricht. (For all the relevant literature of Escher, Romme, and their co-authors or colleagues, see the list of references at the end of this chapter.)

Romme and Escher present a variety of theoretical explanations of hearing voices.
Within *clinical psychiatry*, experiencing hallucinations is regarded as a symptom of a psychiatric illness, notably schizophrenia. One of the reasons why this is negative, is that the construct of schizophrenia lacks scientific validity.

Within *biopsychiatry*, researchers are always looking for physiological causes in the brain. It is well established that certain chemicals (present for example in hard drugs, certain mushrooms or 'strong' soft drugs) may facilitate hallucinations. In such cases, the changes in brain physiology amount to one of the causes of the images or voices, which means their origin is not purely psychological. Also, pharmaceutical medication against psychoses may, ironic though it may seem, evoke hallucinations, and so may Ritalin, a medicine that is sometimes used to treat AD/HD. Some cough syrups contain the substance phenergan, to which children especially may respond with strong fears and hallucinations.

Within *psychology*, hallucinations are mainly linked to a limited capacity to determine whether something really happens or not (reality testing). For young children it is completely normal to have imaginary friends, but later on children typically become more and more able to distinguish between fantasy and reality, unless something goes wrong during the process of development. Bentall and Slade claim that in the course of childhood people slowly but surely develop a theory of mind, in three phases, during which they first realize they have a mind of their own; they subsequently become aware that this also holds for other people, and they finally use this knowledge to formulate assumptions and test these against reality. Ultimately, this leads to the child's ability to distinguish between fantasy and reality. This theory has indirectly influenced psychological views about hallucinations.

Psychologists also link the development of self-awareness, communication, and language to hearing voices. Some believe that young children would generally - more often than older children or adults - attribute an internal monologue, known as inner speech, to an external source. However, there is no consensus about this. The famous developmental psychologist Piaget believed that the origin of inner speech constituted the first stage in the development of language, so that hearing voices could already occur in very young children. However, Russian psychologist Vygotsky believed that inner speech only develops from an exposure to social speech in the outside world. In his view, children will therefore only be able to hear voices by the time they're going to school.

Psychoanalysis holds that hearing voices may be a *defense mechanism* in response to threatening emotions, for instance in connection to a trauma. This was in fact confirmed by research carried out by Marius Romme and Sandra Escher.

According to this tradition, hallucinations may be considered a form of dissociation that is experienced as ego-dystonic (i.e., not belonging to the I). Therefore, having hallucinations is perceived as a symptom of underlying emotional problems.

According to psychoanalysis, another source of hearing voices can be found in the development of the Super-Ego (conscience) or in regression to an earlier, more 'primitive' phase. The treatment of hallucinations depends on the specific source from which they spring.

Some psycho-dynamic *theories* recognize that hallucinations do not necessarily have to be connected to a psychiatric condition. If they are not, hallucinations have a function in dealing with important events in life. They may often act as 'messengers', who can reveal something about the way the person hearing voices relates to others. Among neglected children, they may amount to a compensation for isolation or lack of affection.

Within their own social psychiatric model, Romme and Escher distinguish between several levels within factors that contribute to hearing voices: the *organic level* (the physiological variable), the *individual level* (with psychological, sociocultural, developmental, and spiritual variables), the *social level* (interpersonal factors), and the *societal level* (extra-personal factors). Within their system-theoretical, social psychiatric approach to hearing voices, all these levels are studied separately and their mutual interaction is a focus of research and intervention.

As I said before, social psychiatric researchers Romme and Escher have found a relation between traumas and hearing voices. Seventy percent of people studied by them who hear voices turn out to have experienced one or more – extremely diverse - traumas before their voices manifested.
The main difference with psycho-dynamic theorizing about the origin of hallucinations consists in their greater attention to *social* factors, such as for example may be involved in a trauma.

The consequences of theorizing about hallucinations are enormous. Both in clinical and in biological psychiatry, medication is seen as pivotal.

Psychology is mostly focused on psychological development, and with helping patients cope with their voices.

However, social psychiatry is concerned with the connection between voices and personal problems. In other words, this school is focused on both coping and on understanding the underlying problems.

The approach of social psychiatry as developed by Romme and Escher

From a social psychiatric perspective, Marius Romme views hearing voices as a response to problems. Since the 1980s he has been questioning the bio-psychiatric model. He has met a lot of resistance from fellow psychiatrists because of his claim that in most cases hearing voices is a normal human reaction to an emotional event in the sphere of personal life. Hearing voices occurs in no less than two to four percent of the population, and only for a third of these, does it become so troubling that people start looking for help. Hearing voices occurs about as often among men as among women and it is not connected to age.

Romme's view on hearing voices is related to a general resistance against classifying people with problems in clearly demarcated psychiatric syndromes, a heritage of German psychiatrist Kraepelin. According to Romme, psychiatry has become a prisoner of its own constructs. In his social psychiatric view, phenomena such as hearing voices often reflect situations of psychosocial conflict, rather than some brain defect. Mainstream psychiatry tends to disregard a person's life history and emotional events as factors that may lead to psychological problems. Romme opposes this mainstream disregard with a humanist approach that primarily looks at the individual origin of problems rather than continually stressing psychiatric syndromes.

For instance, hearing voices is often connected to a wide range of incapacitating events in the patient's personal life. Romme and his colleague Escher mention: incest, physical abuse, loss of a loved one, losing authority over one's own children, not being accepted by significant others due to a lack of certain capacities (such as intelligence), lack of self-acceptance related to certain personal characteristics (e.g., homosexuality), living in an aggressive environment without personal control over the situation, etc.

Following research by Sandra Escher and Alex Buis, this also holds for children, who for instance may hear voices as a result of traumatic experiences such as the death of a grandmother, the divorce of their parents, sexual abuse, or the end of a relationship.

The emotions people feel as a result of their situation and experiences have biochemical consequences that may be suppressed by medication, but such suppression simply amounts to a treatment of symptoms and constitutes an obstacle to a true inner healing. People are being estranged from their own experiences and soon run the risk of becoming chronic patients.

Hearing voices is a component of a range of psychiatric diagnoses. Various studies demonstrate that about 70 percent of persons who hear voices report that there is a correlation between the onset of hearing voices and one or more traumatic events.

Obviously, all this also has consequences for treatment. One of the theories about voices and images claims, as I said before, that these carry a certain *message*. Voices often refer to a problem that the person who hears them is facing.

Voices and visions may also be part of a mourning process. Rather than concentrating on the relief of symptoms through medication, it is essential that people learn to deal with their voices in a different way. This also means that they learn to overcome their embarrassment about their voices and talk about them. Also, people who hear voices need to 'own' their experiences, to learn to make their own choices, and thereby to regain control over their lives. This also means that the voices, images, etc. are interpreted within their own philosophy of life. The immediate social environment of family and friends, but also 'fellow voice hearers' or counselors can help them with all this.

Romme and Escher distinguish at least three kinds of relations between voices and someone's personal history. A *historical* relation, such as may occur with traumatic experiences or social-emotional problems, a *psycho-dynamic* relation, in which the voices function as a defense mechanism so that the person can repress the real problem, and a *metaphorical* relation, in which voices manifest in a way that reflects the underlying problems. In general, they hold that voices know the people who hear them very well, and that they're saying things that are relevant to such people. Counselors should realize that the source of their problems, the social situation, has to change, and need to take into account defensive functions and the metaphorical expression of voices.

A variety of behavioral therapies and cognitive methods have been developed to enable persons who hear voices to deal with them in a better way. Cognitive psychology holds that people mistakenly project processes within their own minds to the external world, which means their interpretation of voices is wrong and must be corrected.
Psychoanalysis, analytic psychology, and humanist psychology stress a clear connection with emotional events within one's personal history.
Apart from this, there is a special method, known as the *Voice Dialogue* method, by which one tries to establish a contact with the voices (See Corstens and Romme, 2004).

In order to understand voices and images that are the result of a person's own psychology, it is important to work with concepts such as the *unconscious* or the *subconscious*. Apart from our conscious mental processes (such as our conscious thoughts, memories, etc.), there are simultaneous mental processes that are not directly experienced at a conscious level.

For instance, there is the unconscious processing of information that enables us to do many things automatically and to concentrate on things that really matter. Also, traumatic experiences, negative thoughts or unfulfilled desires can be excluded from consciousness, while continuing to have an impact on a non-conscious level. That we are not aware of a certain process does not mean it is not there (anymore). By acknowledging they are mentally active on many levels at the same time, people who experience impressions without a direct sensory cause, can learn to believe that many of their voices and visions really belong to their own minds and do not come from the world outside.

However, it is possible to take this model too far, namely when people attribute all impressions *exclusively* to their own unconscious and reject the possibility, of, for instance, telepathic impressions out of hand. There is even a current known as *epiphenomenalism*, that regards consciousness as a powerless by-product of unconscious processing. Such an extreme position certainly is difficult to reconcile with an active attitude by which one tries to regain control over one's own life.

In the Netherlands, persons who hear voices have nowadays organized in Stichting Weerklank (Foundation Resonance), which mainly works from a psychological perspective. According to this foundation there is a range of so-called triggers that aggravate the voices, for example:

- feelings: fatigue, stress, anxiety, loneliness, and anger;
- circumstances: negative events, anger or aggression in others, sleeping problems, school examinations, noise or monotonous sounds (shower, fan), conflict situations, being in a new, unfamiliar environment;
- times to which voices can react more than average: when it is dark, during holidays, or at work or school, during visits.

Sandra Escher holds that one should remain aware that a trigger often gives a clue that there is a problem linked to the situation or place.

On the other hand there are also factors that improve the situation, such as 'being physically fit and relaxed, sleeping well, looking for diversions, talking about the voices, asking for help; looking for company, but also looking for rest in solitude.'

Romme and Escher distinguish three phases in experiencing voices. Tilly Gerritsma has elaborated upon these phases in her personal story. We are talking about a:

- Phase of Confusion, that may last for a long or very short time
- Phase of Organization, in which people establish a relationship with their voices, by listening to them and trying to find out their message. During the phase of organization people often learn to deal better with issues like anger, sadness, and loss.
- Phase of Stabilization, in which people reach a balance, accept the message of the voices, and life is seen again from a somewhat broader perspective. There is more to life than just these voices.

Cultural factors

A theory that holds that voices and visions are usually 'normal' psychological responses of people to their situation and life history, also gives room to specifically cultural factors. The inner messages may use images that belong to a certain cultural background. For instance, someone with an Islamic background may hear and see 'djinnis', and a Catholic nun may experience a vision of Jesus or Mary.

By itself, the presence of a certain cultural concept, such as the existence of spirits of the deceased, does not imply that the impressions one may get of them can only have their origin in the person's own mind. This is because some cultural concepts may themselves derive from (interpretations of) primary experiences with an external reality.

Besides, cultural factors naturally play their part in the self-perception of the person having the non-sensory impressions as well. For example, when you are a visionary or a person hearing voices, it makes a great difference whether you are automatically stigmatized as a psychiatric patient, or whether you are seen as someone with shamanic talents or paranormal gifts. In a great number of cultures and religions, from Africa to India and from Peru to Lapland, voices and visions are normally valued in a positive manner as a religious or supernatural phenomenon.

We should realize that (mainly in the West) people with hallucinations have typically been treated in an opportunistic way. For instance, the visions of

Joan of Arc were received positively as long as it was politically opportune to do so, but she was declared possessed by the devil after she had become superfluous. The Holy Inquisition had visionary opponents of the Church condemned to be burnt at the stake because their ideas were too unruly.

Romme and Escher plead for a freedom of inner experience, meaning that people be allowed to develop their own frame of reference within which they can interpret their experiences. It is not at all necessary that this frame of reference match the dominant Western or scientific worldview, as long as the person is dealing with his or her voices and images in a positive way. Within mysticism, shamanism, spiritualism, but also the philosophy of the Dutch thinker Poortman, there is sufficient space for voices and visions as primarily enriching experiences. The researchers also point out that an integration of voices into one's own general outlook on reality lessens the negative impact voices may have upon daily life, and could come to have a positive significance.

Parapsychological phenomena

Parapsychological phenomena are accompanied by inner images or sounds. We cannot say, by the way, that this is always the case. Some phenomena are physical, the so-called *psychokinetic* phenomena, in which the mind exerts a direct influence on physical reality. Psychokinetic phenomena may in fact be accompanied by subjective impressions, e.g., in the case of stigmata, in which a believer may receive a vision of the crucified Christ who lets him or her 'share' in his holy wounds. Afterwards, there turn out to be paranormal wounds (stigmata) on the limbs concerned.

In telepathy and clairvoyance there are 'extrasensory' impressions that can manifest in manifold ways, but are always related to the external world, that is: to physical reality (in clairvoyance) or the inner mind of others (telepathy). Within parapsychology, a great deal of evidence - naturalistic, qualitative, and quantitative - has been collected for the reality of extrasensory perception and its existence normally is no longer doubted by parapsychologists. Sometimes people speak of clairvoyance, clairaudience, etc., to refer to the different sensory modalities that are used to represent paranormal information.

However, within parapsychology, it has been more common to simply talk about *Extra-Sensory Perception* or ESP.

An example of a spontaneous extrasensory impression concerns a vision of a mother who sees the body of her son with the exact wounds of which he has just died. Although she does not know that he has died, her vision turns out to match the facts.

Some people seem to get paranormal impressions so often that they are known as clairvoyants or psychics. During the last few decades, some parapsychologists have doubted the existence of real psychics, while they have continued to take ESP itself seriously on the basis of quantitative experimental research.

Nonetheless, there really is good evidence for the existence of people with a gift for ESP. A few years ago, a book by Barrington, Stevenson, and Weaver was published about the Polish psychic Stephan Ossowiecki. He turns out to have been investigated very thoroughly and it seems quite plausible that he really had far greater psychic talents than average.

Ossowiecki underwent paranormal visual impressions but also many other kinds of sensations. For instance, he got the feeling of choking when he concentrated on the manner in which someone had died (without knowing the cause of death beforehand).

Nevertheless, it would not be very sensible to follow the advice of psychics in an uncritical way. There is no evidence for the existence of *infallible* psychics and all psychics have their own convictions and interests that may influence the advice they give to their clients.

Sheep-like submission may turn a psychic into a sectarian leader warning his disciples of imaginary dangers, keeping them away from mainstream counselors or doctors, or imposing a narrow-minded lifestyle on them.

Apart from extrasensory perception relating to other people (or animals) or concerning the physical world, there may also be perceptions of auras, apparitions of ghosts, or other, spiritual worlds, or communication with the dead or with supernatural and extraterrestrial beings.

To be a little more explicit:

- There is evidence for *auras* in the perceptions of 'naive' persons who never heard or read anything about the subject before they first saw the phenomenon. Young children of 'average' parents constitute an especially important source. The statements of such people seem to match general notions of auras rather well. It seems far-fetched to explain such matches away by mere coincidence.

- Concerning *apparitions*, there are cases in which people saw an apparition of someone they did not know, but whom they were able to identify later on from the images they had seen. Sometimes there is also a paranormal message of a spirit that later turns out to match facts that were unknown at the time, such as the location of a lost will.
Even apparitions of deceased animals sometimes contain paranormal information, e.g., when a dog shows his owner in a vision where his dead body can be found.

- Regarding *images and sounds from other worlds*, there are cases of deathbed visions, Near-Death Experiences, and memories of a spiritual pre-existence. The cases seem to confirm each other in important ways and sometimes involve paranormal information.

For example, a child with memories of a spiritual pre-existence may sometimes mention experiences of his or her parents dating from a period before the child was born, though they had never talked about them in the child's presence. Besides, there are certain elements in these memories that occur much more frequently than we would expect on the basis of childish fantasy, such as the existence of some kind of 'script' or blueprint for the next life, spiritual guidance, and a resistance at the moment the person had to 'descend' into a fetal body.

Near-Death Experiences often occur when there is a flat EEG, i.e., at a moment when according to materialist science, no conscious experience whatsoever would be possible. Furthermore, the person declared clinically dead can in many cases perceive the physical environment and the actions of doctors and nurses, and describe them in detail after resuscitation. These kinds of cases were reported by the famous Dutch cardiologist Dr. Pim van Lommel and his colleagues, such as Peter Fenwick, Sam Parnia, Penny Sartori, and Michael B. Sabom. They constitute a major anomaly for the dominant materialist world view, and one hopes they will get the attention they deserve. Attempts to 'explain them away', such as a recent project by British neurologist Kevin Nelson, are doomed to fail, because they consistently ignore the paranormal side of these experiences.

In the Netherlands, people who had Near-Death Experiences have organized themselves in Merkawah Foundation, a sister organization of the International Association for Near-Death Studies (IANDS).

Deathbed visions of a 'supernatural' reality may be accompanied by heavenly music that can sometimes be heard by others as well. Some patients also see deceased persons whose death they had not yet known about. By-standers may also get visions of unknown spirits who appear to the dying patient and who later on turn out to match specific deceased close relatives or loved ones in physical appearance.

- *Communication with deceased persons* is something that many people actively try to establish, for example through traditional forms of spiritualism, channeling, and instrumental transcommunication, which uses electrical and electronic devices. Besides, there currently is renewed attention to spontaneous contacts with the dead, thanks to the efforts of the formerly married couple Bill and Judy Guggenheim, and others.

Visions or apparitions of the dead which I mentioned before, and other After-Death Communications (ADCs), certainly cannot always be reduced simply to a mourning process. In a great number of cases there really seems to be contact with the dead. Of course, this possibility only makes sense within a theory that takes survival after death seriously.

Finally, it is important that, among others, American psychiatrist Ian

Stevenson and his successor Jim Tucker, and their international colleagues and associates such as Erlendur Haraldsson, Kirti Swaroop Rawat, Dieter Hassler, and Carol Bowman, have given good rational reasons for accepting the existence of *reincarnation*, especially on the basis of their investigations into statements of young children. Such statements form a unity with emotional behavior and a strong identification with the past life, and often correspond to a verifiable deceased personality in great detail, whereas the person in question was unknown to the family before the case started.
These kinds of cases occur everywhere and have been found even in the Netherlands, including by my own team of Athanasia Foundation in collaboration with the Dutch Foundation for Spiritual Development, and the Dutch Parapsychological Institute.

Certain psychological problems and their expression as voices or visions could in theory sometimes be correlated with traumatic experiences from previous incarnations.
In fact, cases have been found in which post-traumatic factors play an important part, such as cases of children who recall a previous life wherein they drowned and who in this life have a disproportionate and inexplicable fear of water, or children who remember how they were murdered and in this life are obsessed by a desire to take revenge on their murderer.

There also are spontaneous images, especially in adults, that seem to correlate with a past life but are really founded on compensatory fantasies. The persons in question probably feel trapped in the banality of their present lives and fantasize about a former existence that would have been much more interesting. Thus, in one case I managed to show that the statements of a retired engineer about a former incarnation as a (doomed) infant on the *Titanic* were almost certainly based on fantasy. The subject supplied many details about life aboard the ship, and so on, that were falsified one by one by documented historical facts.

The acceptance of specifically paranormal images and voices may be part of a new identity, that is often in part defined by culture. Someone may come to see himself as a shaman, as a person chosen by a divinity, or as a psychic.

It seems important to me that people always remain aware of obvious possibilities such as normal internal images and voices. Even psychics, and persons with real memories of previous lives or Near-Death Experiences still remain people with a psychological dynamic and as far as we can tell, there has never been even a single psychic who would consistently have infallible paranormal experiences.

Because of the enormous bulk of evidence for extrasensory perception, I believe it should not even be necessary anymore to prove oneself as a (possible) psychic.
There is also valuable evidence for all kinds of spontaneous paranormal experiences, such as authentic apparitions of the dead or death-bed visions and it is a shame if these are neglected because of a disproportionate amount of skepticism.
Precisely the fact that counselors deny the parapsychological dimension of human life may lead to an exaggerated emphasis on that dimension on the part of the client.
In this respect, it would be good if psychiatrists at the very least learned to show respect for the belief systems of the people who ask them for help and remained open to possibilities that had thus far not been part of their own world view. This might even have a positive effect on the personal growth and ideological development of the counselors in question.

I believe it would go too far to qualify skeptics in general as people who, for 'neurotic' (mildly psychiatric) reasons, shut out anything that does not fit into their ideas, but I do think that the a priori exclusion of paranormal or 'transcendent' phenomena irreconcilable with a materialist world view, seems hardly compatible with a rational - and therefore scientific - attitude toward reality.

Furthermore, it is also important to point out that the development of authentic paranormal 'gifts' may at first be accompanied by all kinds of emotional tests, such as hearing terrifying voices and seeing horrible visions, and even with physical phenomena that are reminiscent of poltergeists. It is tempting to simply view such a phase as a psychosis, but in the context of parapsychology, it may sometimes be more plausible to draw parallels to a period of initiation to which aspiring shamans usually get submitted in non-Western cultures.

Channeling and possession
People have always actively tried to get in touch with higher beings, the souls of ancient ancestors, or deceased loved ones. Spiritualism focuses primarily on communication with the dead, and channeling is mostly a striving for communication with angels, masters or highly developed spirits.
As I have said before, it is good to approach these phenomena with an open but critical mind. Many messages that seem to be transmitted via voices or visions probably are really based - in agreement with the model proposed by Romme and Escher - on inner psychological processes. This normally does little harm, except when people take these messages too seriously and become dependent on them.

Many people believe in a higher self, guide, or guardian angel, who can accompany them on their spiritual path, and as long as they do not lose their earthly common sense, the possible communication with this type of entity via voices and images may be beneficial and promote inner growth. Something like this can be found in this book, in Tilly Gerritsma's story.

There is even some serious evidence for real communication with higher beings, e.g. in Near-Death Experiences and memories of a spiritual pre-existence, but also in the case of spontaneous apparitions of 'angels' with paranormal information that is verified afterwards. British theologian Emma Heathcote-James and Dutch physician Moolenburgh carried out epoch-making research in this field.

A more extreme variant of possible contact with non-physical beings may be found in the possible possession by demons or earthbound spirits of the dead. In this case too, people may hear voices or see apparitions, which are mostly really frightening to them. It is important to take the possibility of inner psychological factors very seriously, if only because the parapsychological evidence for real demoniacal possession (in contrast to evidence for reincarnation) thus far remains very scarce. However, this does not mean that one should not use traditional exorcistic rituals including conversations with the voices (comparable to what is done by the Voice Dialogue method mentioned above) and try to find out what their motives are.

I investigated two young girls who felt haunted by spirits that talked to them and step by step tried to take over their lives. In both cases, there were psychological problems which could explain the voices and visions very well.

In one case, the girl in question was able to realize this, so that integrative hypnotic suggestions could be effective. As a highly gifted child, she could find few suitable friends in her direct environment, so she felt very lonely. She also suffered from tensions between her parents.
However, in the other case, the problem was solved by using a Hindu variation on Roman Catholic exorcism. Because this matched the girl's own personal convictions and those of her mother, the ritual turned out to be very successful. The spirit agreed to leave the girl alone and did not bother her any longer. In this case too there were psychological problems, especially because of the divorce between the girl's parents.

When confronted by the frightening phenomenon of so-called *harming obsession* (an obsessive-compulsive disorder), someone may get the impression that 'demonic beings' are trying to do anything to make their victim carry out violent actions, ranging from wounding someone else to murder. This may be accompanied by obsessive images that seem to come 'from outside'. Scholars have also tried to formulate psycho-dynamic explanations of this phenomenon, but the main requirement is that patients must learn to deal with the obsession, even if for this purpose they use religious ideas about guardian angels and the like.
It is important to note that persons suffering from a harming obsession in reality almost never carry out in reality the violent actions they are so afraid of. In other words, they are not "dangerous psychopaths", but they may suffer a lot under their obsessive imagery and fears connected to these.

Within *transpersonal psychology* considerable attention is given, among other things, to voices and visions in an altered state of consciousness or trance. For instance, they may be part of a spiritual development, such as the one we know from such Catholic mystics as Teresa of Avila, St. John of the Cross, and Hildegard von Bingen, but also from Emmanuel Swedenborg. The person concerned gets in touch with higher forces that under certain conditions are accessible to anyone. Transpersonal reseacher Heery distinguishes three categories of experiences, all of which are accompanied by a continuous learning process with the voices as teachers. The voices would:

- reveal fragmented parts of the self
- take charge of inner development through dialogue
- open channels to a higher level of consciousness

Down with psychiatry?
American psychiatrist Thomas Szasz was profoundly dissatisfied with the way patients were treated in mental health care. He heavily criticized psychiatry in books like *The Myth of Mental Illness* and is often seen as one of the spiritual fathers of the so-called anti-psychiatric movement. Szasz regarded the labeling of clients with psychiatric syndromes as a repressive means to force them to adapt to social and political norms. Similarly, Dutch psychiatrist Jean Foudraine and of course Marius Romme have good reasons to criticize the way that psychiatry has still been functioning during the last four decades.
However, this does not mean that these scholars wish to 'abolish' the entire discipline of psychiatry, but simply that they propose a *reform* that would involve a lot more attention to emotional, psychosocial, and existential factors, and consequently would foster a broad range of psychotherapies. Such changes would be compatible with the social psychiatry defended by Romme and Escher, but also, for instance, with the humanist psychology of Carl Rogers and Abraham Maslow or the ideas of the Austrian psychiatrist Viktor Frankl.

The experiences of Tilly Gerritsma

Tilly's story offers a beautiful illustration of the theory formulated by Romme and Escher, complemented by general parapsychological insights and her own spiritual views. This applies both to the backgrounds of her voices and for their non-psychiatric nature, and also to the successful way Tilly has given her experiences a place and integrated them into a strong personality.

It is to her credit that she wants to share her story with a broad public this way. I hope the project will lead to a feeling of recognition among our readers or else stimulate them to study the work of researchers like Romme and Escher and the activities of Foundation Resonance.

In this context, Marius Romme states (Romme and Escher, 1999): "When we succeed in listening to each other's experiences I think there will be room for surprising and useful discoveries. And it would not be the first time that the study of man can learn something from experiential expertise." (page 39).

Literature

- Barrington, M.R., Stevenson, I., & Weaver, Z. (2005). *A World in a Grain of Sand: The Clairvoyance of Stefan Ossowiecki*. Jefferson/Londen: McFarland & Company.
- Bentall, R. P. (1990). *Reconstructing Schizophrenia.*London: Routledge.
- Blom, J.D.(2003). *Deconstructing schizophrenia; an analyzis of the epistemic and nonepistemic values that govern the biomedical schizophrenia concept*. Boom: Amsterdam.
- Boyle, M.(1990). *Schizophrenia. A scientific delusion?* London: Routledge.
- Busch, M. (1993). *Stemmen horen: wat weten we ervan?* Inleiding Kindercongres Stemmen Horen Amsterdam.
- Coleman, R. (2003). *Herstel, kan dat wel?* Stichting Weerklank.
- Cook, E.W., Greyson, B., & Stevenson, I. (1998). Do any Near-Death Experiences provide evidence for the survival of human personality after death? Relevant features and illustrative case reports. *Journal of Scientific Exploration, 12, 3,* 377-406.
- Corstens, D., & Romme, M. (2004). Praten met stemmen: Over de

Voice Dialogue methode bij mensen die stemmen horen. *Klankspiegel*, *3*, 8-16.

- Dongen, E. van (2004). Als de duivel spreekt laat hij zich niet zien. Over stemmen en cultuur. *Klankspiegel*, 4, 5-8.

- Dorp, S. Van (2002). Kinderen en stemmen. *Deviant*, 32, 32-33.

- Ensink, B. J. (1994) 'Psychiatrische klachten na een misbruik verleden. Een onderzoek onder honderd vrouwen'. *Maandblad Geestelijke Volksgezondheid 4*, 387-404.

- Escher, A.D.M.C. (2004). *An exploration of auditory hallucination experiences in children and adolescence.* University of Central England, Birmingham UK.

- Escher, A.D.M.C. (2005). *Making sense of psychotic experiences.* Proefschrift Universiteit Maastricht.

- Escher, A., Delespaul, P., Romme, M., Buiks, A., Van Os. J. (2003*)*Coping defence and depression in adolescents hearing voices. *Journal of Mental Health.*,*12*,1,91-99.

- Escher, A., & Romme, M. (1998*)*Small talk: voice-hearing in Children. *Open Mind* July/August.

- Escher, A., & Romme, M., (2002). Het Maastrichts Interview voor kinderen en Jeugdigen (MIK*). Tijdschrift van de Vereniging voor kinder en jeugdpsychotherapie, 29*,4, 22-45.

- Escher, A., Romme, M., Buiks, A., Delespaul, Ph., & Van Os, J., (2002).Independent course of childhood auditory hallucinations: a sequential 3-year follow-up study. *British Journal of Psychiatry, 181* (suppl. 43), 10-18.

- Escher, A., Romme, M., Buiks, A., Delespaul, Ph., & Van Os, J., (2002)Formation of delusional ideation in adolescents hearing voices: a prospective study.*American Journal of Medical Genetics*, 114, 913-920.

- Escher, A. D., Romme, M. A., et al. (2003). *Formación de la ideación delirante en adolescentes con alucinaciones auditivas: un estudio prospectivo.* Intervención en crisis y tratamiento agudo de los trastornos psiquiátricos graves. P. Pichot, J. Ezcurra, A. González-Pinto and M. Gutiérrz Fraile. Madrid, Aula Médica Ediciones: 185-208.

- Escher, A.D.M., Romme, M.A.J., Buiks, A., Delespaul, Ph., & Van Os, J., (2002) Kinderen en jeugdigen die stemmen horen: een prospectief driejarig onderzoek. *Tijdschrift van de Vereniging voor kinder en jeugdpsychotherapie*, *29*, 4, 4-21.

- Escher, A., Morris, M., Buiks, A., Delespaul, Ph., Van Os, J., Romme, M. (2004) Determinants of outcome in the pathways through care for children hearing voices. *International Journal of Social Welfare*, *13*, 208-222.

- Fenwick, P. (2004). *Science and Spirituality: A Challenge for the 21st Century*. The Bruce Greyson Lecture from the International Association for Near-Death Studies 2004 Annual Conference.

- Foudraine, J. (1971). *Wie is van hout? Een gang door de psychiatrie*. Ambo.

- Frankl, V.E. (1980). *De wil zinvol te leven: Logotherapie als hulp in deze tijd*. Rotterdam: Lemniscaat.

- Heathcote-James, E. (2002). *Seeing Angels: True Contemporary Accounts of Hundreds of Angelic Experiences*. Londen: John Blake Publishing.

- Honig, A., Romme, M.A.J., Ensink, B.Escher, S., Pennings, M., & de Vries, M. (1998)Auditory Hallucinations: a comparison between patients and nonpatients.*Journal of Nervous and Mental Disease, 186*: 646-65.

- Guggenheim, B., & Guggenheim, J. (1997). *Tekenen van geluk: signalen uit de hemel*. Utrecht: Het Spectrum.

- Kirschenbaum, H., & Land Henderson, V. (red.) (1995). *The Carl Rogers Reader*. Londen: Constable.

- Laudy, Y. (1999). Stemmen horen heel gewoon. *De Telegraaf*, 2 januari.

- Lévinas, E. (2003). *Het menselijk gelaat*. Ambo.

- Lommel, P. v., Wees, R. v., Meyers, V., & Elfferich, I. (2001). Near-death experience in survivors of cardiac arrest: a prospective study in the Netherlands. *The Lancet, 358*, 9298, 2039-2044.

- Moolenburgh, H.C. (2004). *Een engel op je pad*. Deventer: Ankh-Hermes.

- Osis, K., & Haraldsson, E. (1979). *Op de drempel: visioenen van stervenden*. Amsterdam: Meulenhoff.

- Parnia, S. (2005). *What happens when we die?* Hayhouse Inc.

- Parnia, S., Waller, D.G., Yeates, R., & Fenwick, P. (2001). A qualitative and quantitative study of the incidence, features and aetiology of near death experiences in cardiac arrest survivors. *Resuscitation, 48*, 149-

156.

- Rawat, K.S., & Rivas, T. (2007). *Reincarnation: The Evidence is Building*. Vancouver: Writers Publisher.

- Rivas, T. (1990). Intrasomatische parergie: de directe invloed van geestelijke voorstellingen op de fysiologie van het eigen lichaam. (In twee delen). *Tijdschrift voor Parapsychologie, 58, 1*, 9-27 en *58, 2*, 10-25.

- Rivas, T. (1991). Stigmatisatie. *Prana, 63*, 5-12.

- Rivas, T. (1991). Alfred Peacock? Reincarnation fantasies about the Titanic. *Journal of the Society for Psychical Research, 58*, 10-15.

- Rivas, T. (1998). Maya's kwelgeest: Temmigje Rijkse van de Manenburg. *Spiegel der Parapsychologie, 36* (nieuwe editie), *1*, 2-21.

- Rivas, T. (1999). Verscheen Maria in Fatima? *Prana, 115*, 45-51.

- Rivas, T. (2000). *Parapsychologisch onderzoek naar reïncarnatie en leven na de dood*. Deventer: Ankh-Hermes.

- Rivas, T. (2002). Signalen uit de hemel. *Prana, 129*, 63-68.

- Rivas, T. (2002). Aanwijzingen voor het bestaan van een fijnstoffelijk lichaam aan de hand van waarnemingen bij jonge kinderen. *Prana, 131*, 78-83.

- Rivas, T. (2003). *Uit het leven gegrepen: Beschouwingen rond een leven na de dood*. Delft: Koopman & Kraaijenbrink.

- Rivas, T. (2003). *Geen goed leven, geen goede dood: Herinneringen aan Wim*. Nijmegen: Athanasia Producties.

- Rivas, T. (2004). *Encyclopedie van de Parapsychologie van A tot Z*. Rijswijk: Elmar.

- Rivas, T. (2004). Spirituele ervaringen rond het sterfbed van iemand anders. *Terugkeer, 15, 1*, 18-22.

- Rivas, T. (2004). Het geval Alan Sullivan: een bijnadoodervaring met paranormale indrukken. *Terugkeer, 15*(4), 19-21.

- Rivas, T. (2006). Pam Reynolds: psi en een vlak EEG. *Tijdschrift voor Parapsychologie, 1*, 10-13.

- Rivas, T. (2006). Telepathische dromen over overledenen. *Prana, 154*, 29-35.

- Rivas, T., & Dirven, A. (2004) Dankbaarheid bij overledenen. *Tijdschrift voor Parapsychologie, 2*, 16-19.

- Rivas, T., & Dirven, A. (2010). *Van en naar het Licht*. Leeuwarden:

Elikser.

- Rivas, T., & Dongen, H. van (2003). Exit Epiphenomenalism. *Journal of Non-Locality and Remote Mental Interactions, II, 1.*

- Romme, M. (2001). Psychose is bron van ongebruikte kennis. *Klankspiegel*, 2 juni, 9-13.

- Romme, M. (2005). Een kritische beschouwing over de keuze van de diagnose schizofrenie als uitgangspunt van richtlijnen voor de behandeling. *Tijdschrift voor Psychiatrie, 47,* 12, 837-845.

- Romme, M., & Escher, A. (2002). Effectieve en minder effectieve behandelingen van stemmen horen bij kinderen en jeugdigen. *Tijdschrift van de Vereniging voor kinder en jeugdpsychotherapie. 29,* 4, 46-66.

- Romme, M.& Escher, A. (2005). *Managing Distressing Voice Hearing Experiences In Wellness Recovery Action Plan.*(Mary Ellen Copeland edited by Piers Allott.) P.Sefton Recovery Group, Liverpool, UK., p. 114-118.

- Romme, M.A.J. & Escher, A.D.M.A.C.(1987) Leren omgaan met het horen van stemmen. *Maandblad Geestelijk Volksgezondheid 718,*825-831.

- Romme, M.A.J. & Escher, A.D.M.A.C. (1989) Hearing voices. *Schizophrenia Bulletin, 15,* (2), 209-216.

- Romme, M.A.J. & Escher, A.D.M.A.C. (1989). Effects of mutual contacts from people with auditory hallucinations. *Perspectief, 3,* 37-43.

- Romme, M.A.J. & Escher, A.D.M.A.C. (1989) . Stimmen hőren in *Kontakt, Zeitschrift der HPE Österreich, 116.*

- Romme, M.A.J., Escher,A.D.M.A.C. (1990) Effecten van het onderlinge contact tussen mensen die stemmen horen. *Oostland, 2,* 8-14.

- Romme, M.A.J. & Escher, A.D.M.A.C. (1990). Heard but not seen. *Open Mind, 49,* 16-18.

- Romme, M.A.J. & Escher, A.D.M.A.C. (1991). Sense in voices. *Open Mind, 53,* 9 November.

- Romme, M.A.J. & Escher, A.D.M.A.C. (1991).Undire le Voci. *Spazi della Mente, 8,* 3-9.

- Romme, M.A.J. & Escher, A.D.M.A.C. (1993). Hearing Voices (Vertaling artikel uit *Schizophrenia Bulletin* 15-1), *The Japanese Journal of Clinical Psychology,* October 1993, *31,* 2, 65-76.

- Romme, M.A.J., & Escher, A.D.M.A.C. (1999*). Omgaan met Stemmen horen: een gids voor hulpverlening.* Rijksuniversiteit Limburg,

Vakgroep Sociale Psychiatrie.
-        Romme, M.A.J., & Escher, A.D.M.A.C. (1999). *Stemmen horen accepteren: Verschillende manieren van omgaan met stemmen in je hoofd.* Baarn: Tirion.
-        Romme & Escher (2005). Managing Distressing Voice Hearing Experiences In *Wellness Recovery Action Plan.*
-        Romme, M.A.J., Honig, A., Noorthoorn, O., Escher, A.D.M.A.C. (1992) Coping with voices: an emancipatory approach. *British Journal of psychiatry , 161*, 99-103.
-        Sabom, M.B. (1998). *Light and Death: One Doctor's Fascinating Account of Near-Death Experiences.* Grand Rapids: Zondervan Publishing House, 1998.
-        Smit, R.H. (2003). De unieke BDE van Pamela Reynolds (Uit de BBC-documentaire "The Day I Died"). *Terugkeer, 14* (2).
-        Stevenson, I. (1987). *Children who remember previous lives: A question of reincarnation.* Charlottesville: University Press of Virginia.
-        Stevenson, I. (1997). *Reincarnation and Biology.* Londen/Westport: Praeger.
-        Stevenson, I. (2000). *Bewijzen van reïncarnatie.* Deventer: Ankh-Hermes.
-        Stichting Weerklank. (geen jaartal). *Stemmen horen: Wat is het? Wie overkomt het? Hoe er mee om te gaan?*
-        Szasz, T. S. (1970). *De waan van de waanzin: De psychiatrie als voortzetting van de inquisitie.* Ambo.
-        Tenhaeff, W.H.C. (1974). *Inleiding tot de Parapsychologie.* Bijleveld: Utrecht.
-        Tucker, J. (2005). *Life Before Life: A Scientific Investigation of Children's Memories of Previous Lives.* St. Martin's Press.

The experiences and views of Tilly Gerritsma

Why did I write this book?
As a positive individual who used to hear voices, and whose remaining 'voice' soon transformed into a source of inspiration, I want to share my story about the experiences I had to wrestle through. Many people believe hearing voices is part of a disease; meaning that the person in question is, to a lesser or greater extent, crazy. Within other circles, hearing voices is seen as 'paranormal'.

Now, there are two choices you can make. You are either special or crazy after all, because our fellow man does not understand anything of this inner world. Within alternative circles, such as those of holistic healing, natural health, and transpersonal psychiatry, hearing voices is often seen as normal. As an opportunity for growth, a phase of consciousness during which one's own subpersonalities are being analyzed. By externally projecting the (or 'your') voices, you are better able to discover and develop your thoughts, feelings and emotions; it is a possible means of communication between different layers of consciousness. This is normal for many, but for some it may be crazy after all, anything but normal.

Although my voice became integrated very soon, so that I did not really perceive it as a voice anymore, I will still talk a lot about it in this book. Whenever I do so, the voice expresses a certain feeling or thought that I know that does not completely belong to my conscious awareness. Perhaps put in a better way: it is the part of myself that I cannot yet see as a part of my consciousness. In other words, the voice could simply give the deeper aspect of being human, the so-called divine or conscious element in me, an opportunity to express itself in words. This conscious element inside is connected to All that exists, which is often viewed as universal consciousness.

In my perspective, one voice may also represent several feelings or thoughts: just as any human being essentially has many character traits. I can be a good or bad mother, a good or bad friend, a kind or unkind colleague, a good or bad customer.

Why do I insist on sticking to this definition of the voice? I want to break down the difference between being crazy and being normal. The boundaries between concepts like these are so fluid that we can easily flow over into each other's worlds.

The hard thing is to remain standing and this will take a lot of effort. Alternative circles accept the fact that you have to live through certain processes. 'Normal' circles (with some exceptions) do not accept certain processes or do not know how to deal with them. Concerning my 'voice', I now am bold enough to claim that the conscious part of me speaks to me: even in the beginning when I located this part outside myself, but I did feel 'connected' - through a wire - with a deeper aspect of being. Why then did I locate 'the voice', the feeling or the thought outside myself? If I had not done so, I would have run the risk that I (my mind) would have gone astray. In that case, I would have felt so special, because my self would have seemed to know everything. You could say that a voice or guide, a spirit offers some kind of protection by manifesting as a more or less conscious form (a different form) of knowing and being. Your mind can give you insights that derive from a spiritual world so that your understanding of life in all of its aspects will increase. In this area, we should realize that so much is possible; there still remains so much to discover. As we know, testimonies are not always unanimous either. And based on this fact we may suppose as well that a deeper form of knowing can make itself heard and seen in many different ways, depending on your interests and on what you can grasp, what you can absorb at this particular moment as a possible (temporary) truth. After my process, I thus got to know the voice – 'my voice' - as a conscious part of myself that can tell me many things in the field of the transpersonal. It is precisely this part of me that is in touch with the 'supernatural', with the universal field. This field can in principle be accessed by anyone. On a conscious and unconscious level, our souls continuously reach out for this enormous magnetic field in order to understand the 'how' and 'why' of existence. This book tries to unveil some of this by showing what I was confronted with and the coping skills I had to learn as a human being.

The core message
The main message I would like to share with counselors, as someone who has heard voices, is that a person who hears voices can 'shoot' from one dimension (or 'world of feeling') to another. This phenomenon may be related to a psychosocial background that is out of balance. However, it may also happen that a person who hears voices 'shoots through' many facets of the field of universal consciousness, so that his attention does not remain focused enough on the realm of the earthly.

For me, the main thing about hearing voices is that the voice has taught me how to get more insight into my own behavior. Seemingly without effort, I was led, impelled, to get to know myself better and see through myself. This process is taking place constantly and even now I still encounter many steps that I have to make my own. The voice has helped me and is still helping me to become and be a conscious human being.

Questions
Titus and I got to know each other on the internet. By chance, I stumbled upon an article of his that caught my interest and I spontaneously responded to it. That is how we came to send each other numerous e-mails and after I felt we clicked, I asked him if he wanted to write a book with me. A book about hearing voices, or contact with the 'Other Side'. At the same time, I also wrote a very concise overview about hearing voices as seen from the psychological and emotional level, partly because I used to be a member of an expert group (led by Marius Romme, Sandra Escher, and Dick Corstens) that taught me many things. As a researcher, Titus wants to collect as much evidence as possible and I simply tell my own story, my experiences in this area. I asked Titus whether he had any questions for me because my writing style may sometimes be a bit unstructured. I fly from earth to heaven and back, and cover the physical, mental, emotional, astral, spiritual, and universal levels as easily as when I'm peeling potatoes. For me and many others who have tried to reach a spiritual depth, my spiritually inspired texts

are easy to digest. For people who are new to these subjects, my pieces may often seem abracadabra; completely unintelligible. However, I have the same problem when I try to understand a technical subject, or mathematics, medical terminology, etc.

Hearing voices and my personal interpretation
Through *Stichting Weerklank* (Foundation Resonance), working as a voluntary contact person at their aid phone line, I often got to know people with a psychiatric background. I discovered that the boundaries between 'crazy' and 'normal' are often extremely thin. Many people have a gift for mediumship, but they cannot understand their gift in a way that would be acceptable to society, so that their environment often does not understand them anymore. Because I had been dealing intensely with spirituality and had personally lived through all the layers of madness and normality, I understood these people much better. I found that here was an area in which a lot of work still needed to be done to help people progress toward their personal growth, to gain more insight into themselves and in the 'how' and 'why' of existence. This is why in this book I wish to convey a few more insights into what may happen, starting from the notion that the publication of this book and what goes with it is only the beginning of a process that still needs a lot of research and space in order to understand it even better. I will tell about the problems I encountered and the joy I felt when I found out I was no longer all by myself. I naturally realized that a high number of people can learn how to deal with hearing voices if they go for it one hundred percent, with or without the help of counselors who have studied these difficult subjects. To be accepted by your environment, to get a great deal of love and attention, to be taken seriously – these are inevitably connected to mental recovery, which makes living with voices possible. For me it is an enrichment in my life and I cannot imagine that I am so unique as to be the only one for whom such a change is possible.

Titus asked me to tell something about myself and this simple question immediately caused a lot of difficulties. Because: who or what was I? I simply felt like a woman, first of all the mother of my children; at the same time I am connected with a world that is much bigger than my reality here on earth. This is because we can see the earthly realm as a world with a limited level of insight into knowing, thinking, and acting. Just like everyone else, I believe, I am connected with the whole of reality, a world that comprises all the feelings and thoughts that I hardly know yet, let alone that I would understand. And who or what am I in this? What is my share in this? What elements of the things I tell, say, or perhaps claim or believe to be or to know, are mine? By what percentage am I linked to the Other Side, the beyond? And what derives from the beyond; is there really an 'Other Side'? And what has been produced by my subconscious mind? And to what level of my subconscious mind can the Other Side establish a connection? And does this come from the past, the future or the present? And for what purpose?

In order not to get caught up in all these shades of feeling, I simply want to convey the idea that, as human beings, we are not alone. This is my personal opinion and it gives me strength. This is because, in my view, we are connected with everything there is. With the visible and the invisible. There is no death. Our form of being human will end, but, in another form, we will exist forever. We grow, learn, experience, accept, and will shed our form so that we can reappear in another form. Nature tells us so, the animal kingdom tells us so, and mankind also knows this principle. Reincarnation, DNA with all its variants and variables that have not yet or hardly been discovered; continuation of our existence in other dimensions – there still is a lot to investigate. However, in this book I want to focus on the here-and-now, which won't keep me from 'shooting' sometimes from one world into another. Because, from a cosmic point of view,we are living in one world that connects everything to everything else.

Returning to Titus's first question: I am a normal woman who first got acquainted with the phenomenon of hearing voices at a later age in life, who was given this instrument, and learned to deal with it. I have reached a symbiosis and I would not want to miss this for anything in the world. In this book, I describe the way I have done this.

My birth
In November 1953 I was born five weeks early. The dualistic struggle of

wanting to live against not wanting to live, wanting to be versus not wanting to be, was present from the very moment I was born. Five weeks early seemed to indicate a tremendous haste, although I certainly did not feel like starting this life. As a baby, I did not smile to anyone. Not even to my mum and dad, although I was their firstborn and tremendously wanted. I think that, as a personality, I clearly was not into this life very much, whereas my soul, at a deeper level, knew I had to go through with it.

In order to reach a higher spiritual level, I had to be reborn on earth. When I look back at it, I ask myself if the 'better' or conscious half of the world of my feelings was connected to the past or the future. Was my unconscious already capable of seeing the future, and did it know, did it sense, what was in store for me as a human being? Or was it related to causes from the remote past, a preoccupation with my soul consciousness? What part of my personality knew and accepted that I had to be born and what part rebelled against this even then? The need to totally want to accept things turned out to be a big problem even then.

Unfortunately, half a century later, I note that being born, or rather looking at my feelings and emotions with insight, still turns out to be hard.

As said, I was very much wanted as a baby and after having been in an incubator for some time, I grew prosperously. My mother was my safe harbor, because whenever she left the room, I cried out desperately. She had to stay with me, she was not allowed to leave the room. As an infant, I was calm and stayed away from anything that I must not touch. As a toddler I was really clean. The white apron I used to wear as a child for the protection of my clothes, always turned out to have remained white in the evening.

Here again I note, in retrospect, the subject of dominance. They always had to do what I told them to, at first this concerned my mother and later my children, or else I might panic. At a later stage, I also underwent a major influence by religion, upbringing, family, circle of friends, and society. Thus, the cleanliness that characterized me as a toddler, my seriousness and wish to keep everything under control, caused a major breakdown later in life. My subconscious (which I regard as the part of myself that really is more conscious than my waking consciousness and urges me to let that consciousness penetrate into my daily life) will have thought: "It's time for a change."

My childhood years

Our family was growing, so that in time I got two brothers and two sisters. My father was working at an office and my mother stayed at home to take care of the five children. I had a normal childhood. However, I was very sensitive, what they call a *highly sensitive child* nowadays. I would be very cheerful and just one second later I could be depressed if I was affected in a personal way. I also struggled with the normal world view. How on earth was it possible that so much money was spent on space travel, while my fellow human being was starving to death?

My childhood was prosperous, until I entered high school. I found learning rather difficult and although I could have managed the ULO (lower general secondary education), my parents thought it better that I should do the *huishoudschool* (former school for girls who were primarily taught basic housekeeping skills). I was a decent, modest girl. For reasons I still don't understand, at school I was chosen to become the scapegoat. I was completely shut out. There was one girl who made sure that all the pupils were on her side. If they did not support her, she would bully them as well. This negative situation led to my becoming more assertive. But I still remained an adolescent who struggled with humanity and the world we live in.

Perhaps, our situation at home was not very different from that in other families, but I was really troubled by my mother's problems and sadness. My father and mother each had different expectations about their marriage, which weren't always reconcilable. My mother basically had to take care of our upbringing on her own, because my father was completely focusing on his hobbies and interests. Also, she had to try to make ends meet financially, with the money she got from my father. It wasn't possible to discuss this with him. Because I was sensitive and the eldest child, my mother often shared her problems with me, in many respects. People used to keep such things to themselves and she really had to share her sadness with someone.

Thus, my mother shared her sadness, feelings of impotence, and frustration with me and I really felt burdened by the situation. I wanted to protect her and stood up for her, although this naturally did not bring the result I wished for. My brothers and sisters hardly were aware of any of this. Besides, they were younger and not as sensitive as I used to be. They hardly noticed what was going on or perhaps not at all. My mother's wish to do everything on her own (within her own circles) and to learn how to deal with the problems she was facing, undoubtedly had a strong impact on me. Of course, we also need to realize in what period of time all this was taking place. 'Don't tell strangers about your problems' used to be a principle all of us were sticking to. Upon this example, I subconsciously built my own behavior (in terms of shame, stubbornness, and perseverance). I wanted to learn how to deal with the problems I encountered on my path independently, including with regard to hearing voices. And when I wanted to share my problems, I rarely found a person who was my equal, although in exceptional cases this did happen. This situation made me stronger and it helped me put more trust in my inner guide. Because whom else could I approach with my problems?

Adulthood
I followed a course as a nursing auxiliary, met my (now ex-)husband and married at age 21. After I had worked very hard to pay most of the debts we had to incur to buy our own house, it was reasonable to have a child. Four sons were born, all of whom I would like to describe as very sensitive. I thought my marriage was very good, because I wanted it to be so and I wanted to grow old with my husband. In retrospect, I must say that I really had to do a lot on my own. To a certain extent, the same pattern that ruled the marriage of my parents re-emerged during my own marriage. Essentially, I do not want to blame my father, my mother, or my husband for anything, because people can't reach any deeper than their own feelings.

It did cause me a lot of pain, sadness, loneliness, and frustration. To be honest, I hardly ever felt anger, but I did feel sadness. This might be related to former incarnations (and their corresponding stages of consciousness) in which I had already lived through most of this process. My soul consciousness knew that it would not do me any good if I got stuck in it, because I had already undergone this process. The bullying at school, my marriage that had got into trouble; if I think of it, I realize that I hardly suffered under these experiences. You have to take into account that my marriage ended in a pleasant way. We simply had nothing to share anymore, and sexually our marriage had also run dry. We remained good friends, which of course was very pleasant for all of us. However, before we had reached that point, apparently, my life was building up to a climax (as if this was only natural or predestined) so that I started hearing voices.

At the age of 26, I gave birth to my eldest son, Bart. Bart was born three weeks early. He was a sweet, cheerful and extremely active little boy. Bart was really social, a very sensitive child, but also rather domineering. Although I consulted the RIAGG (Regional Institute for Ambulatory Mental Health Care) at an early stage, they did not notice anything peculiar about the child. He just was very active, and that was the only thing they could tell me. Only later on, when his behavior escalated during puberty and he started using drugs and got involved in petty theft, they diagnosed him as having Attention Deficit (Hyperactivity) Disorder.

Bart dragged his brother with him into his negative circle of friends and my third son was also vulnerable in this respect. My general practitioner advised me to throw Bart out of my house. I couldn't handle the situation, and my husband was even worse at it. He literally shut the situation out by putting on a headphone so that he wouldn't have to be present. Our family, and especially myself, were at risk of going under. We had to choose between one particular child and our whole family. This choice was very difficult for me.

At first, I did not want to follow the advice of throwing Bart out. There must be some way to keep the family together! I just couldn't let go of my child whom I loved so much and hand him over to strangers. Hadn't I done my utmost to help him out?

After I had done everything I could for 15 years, it was clear something had to change. For me, throwing out my own son was a tremendously traumatic experience. Perhaps, at a subconscious level, I felt that I had failed (I mean psychologically), although at the same time, I knew I had done everything I was capable of.

In the meantime I'd survived on Seroxat, an anti-depressant prescribed by my physician. Seroxat made my emotional life less intense, but of course it did not solve anything. In the long run, I decided that this medication didn't work anymore. Depression showed up again, whereas the medication was meant to do the opposite. "By chance" I met a therapist with an alternative background. We both were doing a course in painting watercolors. "Would you do something for me?" I asked her. "Could you give me some energy so that I will hold on?" She told me she could. And that is how I got acquainted with the so-called paranormal circuit. Although this field had never appealed to me, I had reached the end of my strength. The world of the paranormal struck me as really strange. They claimed they could foresee the future and predict illnesses and so on. Now how could that be healthy? I had absolutely no experience with the paranormal and what I heard about it did not appeal to me. Years before, my mother-in-law and sister-in-law had visited some kind of soothsayer. Someone who knew things about you and could see into the future. She told them that my sister-in-law was quite ill and that the doctors were wrong about her. It turns out, my sister-in-law did die young after an operation and several treatments, years later, but did she really have to know? I found this extremely hard to swallow, especially because my sister-in-law never accepted her approaching death and passing over. That was one of the reasons I was not exactly pleased by the paranormal. On the other hand, mainstream medicine was stuffing me with pills, which after a while did not even work anymore. I had to do something and that is why I tried the alternative field. I had to choose between swimming or drowning, fighting or fleeing, and I chose to fight.

Hearing voices
Looking back at it, I clearly started hearing voices after a traumatic experience. The first time I heard voices, or to be precise one single voice, it happened during a state in between my waking and sleeping consciousness. In the morning, I also heard (and I still hear) inspirational voices, while my

mind still needed to wake up. Maybe it's related to the fact that in both cases I'm free of thoughts so that 'they' can influence me. Or it may also be that in this state of mind I automatically connect to a deeper level of consciousness. Later on, I realized that I somehow needed to attune my mind, concentrating on a relevant problem or question so that they could deal with it. Or that I had to automatically reach a calm state of mind of surrender and try not to be dominated by feelings and emotions, so that I could become receptive to certain insights.

During these difficult times, in which I had to let go of my beloved child under such unnatural circumstances, I was really losing control.
On the other hand, I received the help that I needed so badly and that would change many things.

Months before the decision that was so difficult for me, I was already completely exhausted, both physically and mentally. At the time, I was working as an auxiliary nurse during night shift and during the day I was sleeping a lot. This urge to sleep, trying (needing?) to find rest, to withdraw from daily life, increased more and more, even when I wasn't on night shift. One afternoon, I was lying in my bed again. It happened just before I fell asleep. Something that sounded like the English word FAITH was being said very loudly at my left ear. I immediately felt euphoric and I thought joyfully: "They have come to help me, I don't have to do it on my own anymore." I ran for the dictionary to check whether I had heard the word correctly and went back to bed in a state of euphoria. Shortly afterward, when I had almost fallen asleep again, I heard someone say TRUST loud and clear. It was a female voice and it sounded as if the voice was determined to make me understand what she was saying. It was as if somebody were standing next to me, but of course I didn't see anyone. I immediately interpreted the voice as that of a helper, a guide, an entity, and of course somebody from a higher realm. Because only such a guide could help me, or so I thought. In those days, I was seeing the therapist I had met at the watercolor painting course. She gave me a paranormal healing, which really led to a fantastic result. I stopped having cold feet, had plenty of energy, and could handle life again. In the same period I started hearing the voice and I immediately saw a connection to the Other Side. I had heard a lot about it by that time, and my therapist was also connected to it, so I surely was experiencing the same thing.

I have no idea what the therapist was doing to me, what it was that she was healing and opening at the same time. However, it did mean (I felt it did) that I ended up in another class and that I had to start at the bottom again. My therapist hardly ever talked about the paranormal. She told me hardly anything and I rarely asked her any questions about it, because I knew almost nothing concerning this field. And I still found it a bit frightening as well. What on earth did they know 'up there'? Could they see through me just like that? It really is horrible if you cannot hide anymore. Don't forget I was far from perfect. And what did my therapist know? Could she also see through me? Therefore, I wisely kept my mouth shut, but on the other hand I did feel some curiosity regarding this area. My therapist recommended a book by Louise L. Hay, *You Can Heal Your Life*.
Very interesting, but was all of it true? Many things were happening to me. It seemed as if thousands of feelings, thoughts, and images were sweeping over me and overwhelming me. One day, when I revealed everything that was happening to me to my healer, she told me that nothing surprised her anymore. She'd had so many experiences already. At the same time, I didn't know how to handle it.

We didn't continue to talk about it, and it may also be possible that it simply frightened me too much.
Besides, I noticed that her life was not exactly perfect either, which made me doubt her abilities somewhat. Her healing method consisted of 'magnetic' paranormal healing, which turned out to be helpful for me, so that I could go on again. But in other respects, it seemed I had to find my own way again. Through dreams and visions, I got in touch with previous lives that explained why I liked or disliked someone. I received an image in which I was walking along a beautiful paved street together with my husband (possibly in the eighteenth Century). (Did they already have cobblestones in those days? Or had I mixed up images and feelings from different lives?)
I was dressed in a long skirt with a short jacket and my husbandwas wearing a hat. I was holding a small parasol in my hand. I was a cheerful and

51

spontaneous woman, my husband was very serious. We entered some kind of pharmacy; my husband seemed to be the pharmacist.

In another lifetime, I'd been a witch and I was burnt. In yet another life, I had to deal with jealousy and I ended up killing my husband who was cheating on me with numerous other women.

In yet another life I was living in England, in a gorgeous cottage. I saw how I was being raped by several men, after which I was murdered. During my present life time, I met these men again. I knew why I was married to my husband, why we had to - or were allowed to - let each other go, and what kinds of relationships I'd had with men and women in previous lives.

Proofs? No, no proof, but the images and feelings I got to see, ensured that I started to understand the world better and to see it in another light. It was my truth, my (temporary) knowledge, but not anything more than that. It ensured I remained standing upright and could get on with my life.

Years later, when I started reading the books by Marius Romme and Sandra Escher, I realized I fitted perfectly into the model they describe in their book *Accepting Voices.* In this model, they distinguish different phases people who hear voices have to pass through. I had obviously passed through the first phase, the phase of confusion. There was a lot going on in this period that was enriching my mind but also confusing me. The phase of confusion took at least several months. To be honest, the real confusion already started before this period. I had a burn-out and it was only after my burn-out that what psychiatrists call the phase of confusion began. I would prefer to call this period my *awakening*. Awakening, being born again, meaning that you have to learn everything (all over again). Just like a baby who has to learn everything from scratch, I had to understand the other world better, in other words: at a deeper level of consciousness. The second phase, the phase of organization, essentially began immediately after I'd heard the positive voice for the first time. After I had slowly learned to let go of my fear (a certain amount of fear has a constructive impact and is necessary within human consciousness) the phase of organization had come within my reach.

These two phases are followed by the stabilization phase. The first two phases really go together because, among other reasons, my positive 'voice' guided me through my process of getting to grips and dealing with the realm of the 'Other Side' from the very beginning. But stabilization also made itself felt now and then, from the very start. The element of hearing, of sensing at a deeper or more conscious level of feeling, knowing, and being, was my priority from the very beginning. So, on one hand, I took on a dependent attitude; I wanted to hear and listen to anything the voice needed to tell me. At the same time, I had to be morally sound if I wanted to receive messages that would be pure. The desire to understand; trying to be morally sound; getting to know and recognize my personal world of feelings through introspection and reflexion, certainly helped me with all this. Therefore, there is essentially no absolute boundary between the phases, but they can partially happen at the same time.

During the phase of confusion I underwent the following experiences:

- I heard a voice.
- Later on, I heard several voices.
- I often felt an energy that passed through me.
- I had to deal with a negative energy.
- I had to deal with dreams.
- I saw images that couldn't be seen with the normal eyes.
- I had to deal with energy forms (thoughts and streams of feeling: entities?).
- I heard sounds nobody else could hear.
- Never alone again.

1. I heard a voice in English, and after a while, I tried to understand what it was saying: Wake up, there is more between heaven and earth, you are not alone. Why was it talking to me in English? To demonstrate that it really was something special, something I really needed to listen to. I had to make an effort, it was not my everyday language. My curiosity was being aroused.

2. Later on, I heard several voices that were all shouting at the same time. Information that I wanted to have but also information I had not asked for was crossing my mind. I ran the risk of going mad. I realized (I was told by my guide, my spiritual coach or a deeper layer of consciousness) that I had to learn to shut off. I was as open as possible and I let everything pass through me. This clearly was not what I was supposed to do. I learned that my will was a fundamental power through which I was able to decide for myself what I did and did not allow to enter into my inner world. After all, on earth people also choose their own friends, what they want to eat, what kind of clothes they want to wear. You have the same kind of choices when you are in contact with other dimensions. I do not interpret all the voices I heard in that period as independent spirits (little personalities outside myself), but I see some of them as my own feelings and thoughts that were flooding me at that moment.

3. I often felt an energy that passed through me. During the phase of confusion I was helped by an energy that passed through me and temporarily helped me with my confusion of feelings and emotions. Some kind of serenity descended onto me (while my problems were being covered or transformed?) so that it seemed as if all my cares and problems were over. They were still there, but far away, they didn't bother me anymore. I also heard (and felt) that I was given support so that my emotional life could bear and undergo everything (something similar often happens during the dream phase). Later on, I would need to stand alone, on my own feet. That's why I noticed it, whenever the 'medicine' - which can best be compared to an enormous dosage of rest, love, primordial power - was disappearing from my body. Or was it temporarily dissolving to resume its own level within the subconscious again? Whenever this happened, I grew more anxious and I was confronted by my feelings and my thoughts. I have no idea what was happening when the primordial force manifested in me. However, I was strengthened by all the confusion I'd been through and could face life again. Whenever I risked falling back into depressive thoughts, I was told lovingly but admonishingly: "Come on, girl, you can do it. Consciously and subconsciously you're creating everything yourself and consciously and subconsciously you are attracting everything that is happening to you."

I learned to go toward the pain. Some people believe that pain is good, but I think this means giving the feeling of pain too much credit. I did notice, though, that there is a message to pain. By going toward the pain (or anger, sadness, impotence, insecurity) the feeling dissolved, to a certain extent. It was only then that I could see the deeper layers of my feelings. I could analyze the feelings and emotions that were annoying me without judging or condemning them. I like to compare this energy with some kind of omniscient father or mother assisting me like a child on my path through life. Every child is supposed to become an adult and in that sense I had to let go of my childhood so that I could stand on my own feet. After all, the child needs to become an adult, a father or a mother, and cannot remain a child for all eternity.

4. I had to deal with a negative energy and that was a very strange experience. One afternoon, I was resting on my bed again, because I was physically and mentally exhausted. Suddenly, I felt an energy in my body of which I had not been aware before. I was in a hypnagogic state of mind. I had not been thinking about anything, but all of a sudden I was startled by something and I was fully awake immediately. A warm current, an agreeable stimulation, took possession of my body. It slowly crawled from my back to my breasts. It was as if I was looking at this process as an observer and at the same time I remained able to feel what was happening to my body. I felt the warmth and the tickling and, to be honest, at first I really liked it. It isn't that unnatural either, when you have been sexually dissatisfied for years. Simultaneously, I was watching everything that was going on "down there" and I felt how the energy kept descending more and more to my lower body. When I realized that this form of energy was trying to take physical possession of me, I decided to stop it. On the inside, I was yelling: Stay away from me, I don't want this! Get lost! I was literally crossing my legs and tightening my muscles until I felt that nothing could pass through anymore. My body was completely locked up. The energy left and he or 'it' never came back.

Why did this happen? My spiritual guide or my subconscious mind told me that as a human being I had a natural need for sexuality. For years, my husband had barely touched me. Because of my mediumistic personality, I was automatically attracting energy waves that were connected to sex. My body was confronted by an immaterial being that wanted to experience bodily warmth or sex. I was looking from above at the scene that was developing below. I had ended up in the middle of a situation, but this was only partially true, because I still had an overview of it. To a certain extent, I could approach it rationally and I saw that I was being physically and emotionally attacked by the astral or mental world. That way, I was confronted by my own subconscious feelings that were manifesting in me, and it was a fact that I had opened myself up to this.

In my view - and I'm not saying that I fathom the depth of all this - being a medium means that I have a certain sensitivity, through which I can connect to the universal aspect of being. I do not mean to say that these frequencies of feeling are always pure, that's a different story. It is also related to the fact that I turn my attention to my inner being, which could also be called the beyond. In this context, the beyond is the source that can permeate everything so that it may also be sought outside my own self. The domain beyond my emotions, beyond my psychological field, beyond spirituality may also be seen as the universal aspect of being human. Therefore, to be a medium does not mean to be good or bad. It may be seen as a gift, but also as a handicap. In my case, I knew from the first time I started hearing voices (which could have been my surfacing subconscious) that I had to adopt an attitude to them which was as pure as possible. Now that I had opened up, in principle anything could pass through me, approach me. My attitude or attunement was and continues to be very important. Because what does my *I* really want? The deeper part of my I-consciousness was not and is not exclusively focused on the earthly frequency of feeling.

It was important to become aware of my, often subconscious, feelings. I personally had the power to open up to them or to seclude myself from them. Consciously and subconsciously I could attract anything to me, but I also could, and I effectively learned how to, distance myself from anything.

5. I had to deal with dreams. For my entire life, I've always dreamed a lot, but I never gave it much thought. Only after I had opened up to everything that was happening, to what was going on inside me, did I learn to understand this world better. Through the dreams and images that I got during the day, I realized that my marriage was not good. "Not good" is essentially an inadequate qualification. I would rather say that we were both through with our relationship and that each one of us was allowed to continue on the paths we had to walk. It is related to past lives (older or more or less unconscious frequencies of feelings), to karma (cause and effect) that was being solved. For me, this explanation was sufficient and my ex-husband and I could go on with our lives. Also, I was shown through dreams and images that I shared several lives with a man whom I had met at that particular moment. From a psychological point of view, this is not very odd, because I didn't get enough attention and love. What was strange about it, was that at first I had not noticed the man in question, and that I had not been in the least attracted to him. It was only later on, through the dreams and images projected to me out of the blue, that I saw several lives with him passing by and I understood my sensitivity and my connectedness to him. Past, present, and future got mixed up with each other, and I didn't know how to separate them. We did have an emotional bond (which of course was felt more by me than by him), a beautiful relationship of trust. We were both attuned to the same frequency whenever we were striving for the same goals, but that was all there was to it. My husband's feelings and my own feelings were not mutual. And even on this point, I did receive an explanation which was acceptable to me. My husband and I were coming from different frequencies of feeling (past, present, and future) and therefore we couldn't understand each other emotionally. When you realize this, it is something very natural, although most people usually will not think about it so deeply. For me, it offered me an opportunity, a broader framework, to deal with my grief.

I was able to go on with my life and I also had to go on. We were divorced now and I really understood that this was the best outcome for the development of both of us. For myself, my ex-husband, and even our children. In yet another dream, I saw the image of a man who was going to visit me the next day. His luscious hair was the first thing that had called my attention. It was very amusing that the same person was really standing before me in real life later on. In yet another dream, I was shown a prophetic vision that materialized afterward. In my dreams, I often received warnings for things that were happening to my children (your son is smoking cigarettes or pot, he took some money from your wallet, etc.). I was often told in my dreams (via metaphorical images) what was going on with the person in question so that I would be able to make some peace with it.

6. I saw images that couldn't be seen with the normal eyes. I saw a man standing in front of me who really wasn't there. I knew (or it was my interpretation) that he was a temporary connection from a previous life. I saw flashes of children who weren't there. Amusing, but also strange; I wasn't supposed to do anything with it, and I can't explain it either. Only in a few instances did it have a certain meaning which was only made clear to me later on. At times, I saw a phantom flashing by. On other occasions, I saw all kinds of energy forms that continuously changed their shape and color. I wouldn't know what it all meant or conveyed.

7. I had to deal with energy forms (thoughts and streams of feeling: entities?). Although at first this was very confusing, it soon became part of reality (a natural possibility) that after a while was integrated into my life. I received greetings from people who'd passed away, loving messages, and on rare occasions a loving request: "Please, pass this on to..." There were fragments from contacts I'd had before, in previous lives. Sometimes I noticed that this could offer some consolation to someone, but that was all I was able to do with it. I really didn't want it; it made me feel insecure and I didn't feel like it. The point is I didn't *see* any spirits or entities; my feelings were simply influenced directly. And while I noticed that the person felt moved by what I was saying, I didn't like it myself and I didn't want to get in touch with the hereafter this way. Although I know that many people draw some comfort from the fact that you can get in touch with deceased loved ones, I do not regard this as my personal path. From my perspective, every being and spirit continues to grow in consciousness. The wish to keep on communicating with a loved one may also impair this spirit (or layer of consciousness) in his or her development; he or she is in a way kept back in this field of consciousness, and this is also true for the people who are searching for this field consciously or subconsciously.

8. I heard sounds nobody else could hear. I heard the phone ringing in my mind, and just a few moments later, the phone actually started ringing. While meditating, something was added to my inner world; some feeling was triggered and activated in me. Something outside or inside myself was calling my name and I automatically listened to what it was telling me. Although in the beginning these experiences were a bit confusing, I soon underwent this form of communication as an enrichment. Nine out of ten times, after I woke up, I used to get the feeling that something was being put inside me (that I was being linked to the deeper layers of my soul): "Come on, it's time to get to work again." The guide (the deeper layers of my being) knows how far I've come in my development, what point I've reached, what I still need to learn, what I need to do once more, because I still haven't mastered it enough, etc. Some thought is activated in me and I start working on it. Sometimes, I used to go too far in this process. My guide led me back to the right path so that I didn't get lost in the enormous amount of information that was available to me (more about this below, where I discuss 'round thinking'). Whenever my subconscious mind awakes me, I'm immediately lucid and start doing the mental work. Of course, it is I who takes on this attitude, turning my attention inside, but I know that it contains a deeper knowledge, which essentially transcends my earthly frequency of feeling. It is there that I can find my personal development and nowhere else. Although I naturally do need the external triggers, the answer to the question what I could or could not do with it, can be found within myself. What's striking about this is that I always used to suffer from a lousy morning mood and always needed time to get going. I don't anymore.

9. Never alone again. Although my first contact with hearing voices was positive, it also brought along an enormous fear. What did they know about me? Could an entity, a spirit know everything, see everything, even read my plans and thoughts, my negative feelings about what I was and was not doing? I could not hide; 'they' could watch me and simply enter my inner world.

'They' or 'it' knew me better than I knew myself. Fortunately, there always was this positive voice to shake me awake. *Do you really think that a higher spirit endowed with more awareness, a higher consciousness would want to embarrass you? That they would like to pull your leg or harm you? Only man or a lower consciousness (spirit, entity) would do so. If we condemn your actions or warn you, it will always happen out of love. It will never be destructive. A warning or insight will manifest in such a way that it will increase your understanding. That way, you will always be able to think deeper and deeper, to sense how things are, through which a universal knowing will arise.*

This reassured me again. If you think of it, it really makes no sense to be afraid. Because what, in heaven's name, did I possess that others did not? Essentially, every person carries all feelings inside. On one occasion you feel (even if only for a second) superior, on another occasion you feel like the greatest sucker that walks the earth. The voice always made me keep my feet on the ground, just like the many books I read at a later stage, so that if necessary, I could be reminded of a certain sentence. "If you think you have reached perfection, you have not. Life is one big learning process. Human beings cannot really think (because our thinking is purely focused on life on earth)," were messages that have helped me enormously. 'The voice' as a positive feedback, support, and anchor, hope, faith, and love quickly alternated. I ask myself to what extent we may speak of a cosmic or universal inspiration here, or of a certain kind of consciousness that I have made my own in the course of years. "Stay in control of yourself and you control the world," was also a line that seemed to be made for me. Similarly, for any person, there are aphorisms with a certain emotional value that seem apt for him or her at that specific moment.

Whenever I had read something, had let something sink in, it appeared as if I was being plugged in into a big computer so that the right file came to me when I, apparently, needed it. On the other hand, I also think that I had already been linked to this computer. Everything I learned from 'the voice' or my deeper inner world, turned out to be reflected by the contents of all kinds of books later on. It is as if I was automatically connected to the universal channel and really did not need to read any books anymore. However, because I'm a quite incredulous and very fearful human being, the books gave me the confirmation I really needed.

After having recovered from the shock that I would never be alone again, I even found the idea quite agreeable.

During the phase of confusion and also during the phase of organization I was mainly confronted by my own thoughts, feelings, and emotions that got hold of me. When I first heard a voice say *Faith* and *Trust*, I thought that I was really special for a while. I belonged or was going to belong to the circles of paranormal people.

But was I really happy with this? I was being overwhelmed by a thousand and one feelings, running the risk of going crazy. Obviously, this feeling of being special later disappeared, but it did untie certain feelings in me. I went through:

- euphoria: I was very special. The therapist/healer I was seeing did not correct this feeling.
- depression: I didn't dare talk about all the things I was experiencing and going through mentally. (the therapist in question was leading a personal life that I did not exactly approve of. Love and unity were sometimes hard to find.)
- confusion: What is happening to me?
- loneliness: I could talk to no one, and even alternative circles only told me what they could or were allowed to say.
- anger: Why did I have to experience this, why did it happen to me?
- sadness: Why couldn't I express myself to my partner, family and friends?
- fear: What did the voice know about me, was I completely transparent to the voice?
- insecurity: What mistakes did I make?
- surrender to a higher power
- trust in a higher power

Phase of organization

During the second phase, the phase of organization, the voice and I had reached an agreement. I listened to the voice, because I noticed that it helped me with my process: how I had to deal with sadness. Because at the time sadness was the main, dominant feeling (although in essence it may be reduced to fear). Not being able to accept what I saw as reality in my existence. Through a process of internal communication, I increasingly started to know and recognize myself, my thoughts, feelings, and emotions. I think that many feelings arise from the unconscious. Nevertheless, some feelings could derive from an extraterrestrial realm, or the beyond, the universal field, if you prefer. I couldn't tell to what percentage I'm connected to the beyond. If you realize that through the years I read many books that appealed to me, and on which I put my hope, faith, and trust, you may say that this undoubtedly enriched the experience of how I take in and undergo things. In my view, the beyond was continually being integrated into my personal life. You always continue to learn (as in a regular course) and I made everything I was learning (what was coming to me) my own. After that, the next process is started naturally, depending on your personal will. We start with a new layer for which the deeper part of yourself is naturally addressed as well. By now, the phase of confusion won't adopt such extreme forms any more, so that you can live through the process without any major shocks. You know what's going on and what needs to be done and you know you have to adopt the attitude of a pupil time and again.

If we realize that man really knows everything already or at least has the potential of knowing, and at the same time can be in touch with the universal aspect of being, it seems this is a beautiful field of investigation.

During the phase of organization I had to deal with the following issues:

1. Who or what is the voice?
2. In dialogue with the voice
3. With whom do I want to collaborate?
4. What do I want to know?

1. Who or what is the voice?
I experience 'the voice' as a domain of feeling (an entity, a guide, if you like), a coach helping me during my process of developing as a human being. The voice has its own subjective world that represents a certain degree of consciousness. At the same time, the voice is able to get in touch with a still higher or deeper consciousness. You may call it a higher or more conscious

domain of feeling within the universal field, the all-encompassing field of knowing, feeling and being. In my view, in the other world there is a hierarchy similar to the one on earth. A baby needs help from its father and mother, it even wholly depends on them. An infant, toddler, and child still need their father and mother. But even the adolescent, the young adult, and the adult, even though they are independent, all need another human being to learn, to develop, to ask, to give, and to share.

It is possible to recognize the same principle at a cosmic level in positive and negative energies that we experience as entities, spirits, extraterrestrial life, energy spheres or orbs, contact with the field or the universal aspect of being. Good and bad, conscious and unconscious, they are all part of the universal consciousness that always continues to deepen and expand. Of course, there is also your own voice(s) that you recognize as a kind of warning, memory, reflection of a certain feeling.

2. In dialogue with the voice

When I had recovered from the first euphoria and shock, I began to directly communicate with the voice. (I first heard one voice, only later on there were several voices, and it was hard to communicate with them, because they got mixed up with each other.) In the beginning, I did not know if it was my inner world, my thoughts, wishes, and emotions, or if it was really coming 'from outside'; my spiritual guide. This related to the fact that the voice was integrated into my consciousness fairly soon. This meant I still had to learn to feel what subtle feelings were coming 'from outside' and what feelings could be regarded as the result of my own mind. What was mine and what belonged to the beyond (a deeper consciousness)? It still was a major job to find out, but the positive voice was helping me in the process. It really wasn't that important as long as both of us (myself and my guide) were striving for one and the same goal. I was learning more and more when I was really being inspired and when I was functioning out of my own strengths. Whenever I was being helped or inspired, everything went perfectly. I was talking fluently and I knew exactly when I had to say something and how I had to say it. This does not mean everything was pure, because my own consciousness was partly interwoven with 'the beyond' (the subconscious). Because I'm a very emotional human being, in those days I often subconsciously created a blockage that could not be broken down by positive energies. I was stuck in sadness, insecurity, fear, and so on. They also tried to change this cosmically, so that I was learning to expand my level of consciousness from the beginning of my universal cosmic 'education' (the first year of high-school, so to speak). Unfortunately, it took me many years before I noticed that I wasn't that depressed anymore, that I could handle the outside world better.

A dialogue with the voice needs to be somewhat fluent. Whenever I'm being disturbed by too much negativism, by feelings and emotions that are too dominant, they can't get through. I'm being overly influenced by personal circumstances; my feelings are excessively dominating my consciousness.

Painting

Right from the start, I wanted to paint, perhaps I was being inspired by my guide to do so. I started with a watercolor painting course, but I couldn't express myself enough with it. I had reached the stage of my life in which I had to evict my son and I suffered intensely because of it. I literally painted away my sadness, my anger and frustrations. At the same time, there always was some light in my paintings, because I knew I was being helped, supported, guided, and coached. But the 'junk', what I would consider my negative unconscious later on, repressed feelings, had to be dumped. In my first painting, inspired by the voice and my belief in the beyond, I had painted so much faith, hope, and love (color and shape), that nobody discovered my intense sadness in it. My painting was first and foremost related to psychological processing. Feelings, thoughts, and emotions that I depicted, so that they could be processed and released. My feeling activated me to make a number of paintings.

I once made a painting that I didn't like very much. I thought the colors weren't great, but... it had to happen that way. Strangely enough, it was precisely this painting that people found exceptionally beautiful and powerful. It is interesting to note that my paintings became ever more spiritual, after I had made several of them. At that moment, I had hardly taken a look at spirituality and still I was painting the beyond, death, life and reincarnation. My last paintings represented God (the All) and I painted them in gold. I didn't even dare sign them, that's how 'sacred' they were. Of course, nobody saw that it was God and I naturally didn't tell anyone either. They would have thought I was 'insane' and I didn't want to be seen that way. Of course, after God, I'd reached the end of my artistic journey. Because you can't go any higher than God, can you? When I started studying spirituality later on, I noticed that my subconscious had painted something of which I'd hardly been aware as a human being. My subconscious had revealed something, through the voice, to which I was connected by nature, but which I hadn't integrated into myself yet. I found it very amusing to encounter this layer of consciousness in various books later in life.

Music

After this period of painting, I started working with music. It still was a question of psychological processing. I danced my sadness away with beautiful movements, with raw 'violence', and with a stream of tears that seemed to be endless. I was super-sensitive. A single song, a remark, a beautiful flower, a tree, the air, an animal... At that moment in time, I could be touched by almost anything, as long as it established a contact to my inner consciousness. After I had finally stopped crying – I had bottled up negative emotions for years, so there were many tears to shed – I was ready and I could listen to music in a normal way.

Writing

The third type of psychological processing consisted of writing. Third time lucky, so I wasn't ready yet. However, this time it was psychological processing that I was getting through, that I was taking in, that I had to exclude, filter, coordinate, transform, let go, and so on. This writing started during the phase of confusion, and it persisted through the phase of organization to finish during the phase of stabilization.

I learned very soon that I also wanted to verify what I was receiving. After all, my I was still present and I wasn't a completely passive person with no opinion of my own. I checked the 'difficult words' that I received in the dictionary and I wanted to write them down only after I had done so. The way the words were used was always correct and when I incidentally decided that a certain word really was too difficult, they industriously (at least, that's how I interpret it) searched for another word. My wish was their desire, if I may say so. 'They' (a deeper part of myself) didn't want to lose touch with my present I, or in other words: my daily (household) self still had a say in how things went, and they really took (or had to take) this into account.

During the transition between the phase of confusion and the phase of organization I got rid of anger, sadness, impotence, aggression, and fear, through my writing. I was angry because I was angry. I had shut out a whole range of feelings that I didn't want to recognize, because I found them utterly bad, under the influence of my upbringing, environment, culture, and society. I was told to describe myself as a house and I did so many times. Often, I also described the neighborhood, the environment, the street, and the whole village. This was a fantastic therapeutic way of getting more insight into my feelings that I had hidden all my life. I looked at my house as an observer and talked about everything I was seeing. I was there, I was in and out again, I remained at a distance and got closer, I switched from positive to negative and back.

I feel I was dealing with some kind of psychologist from the beyond who advised me to write about my feelings: a therapeutic process to get more insights into my inner feelings and experiences. The stories I wrote symbolize my feelings and my emotions, my impotence, but also my strength and determination to get to know myself better. I did this in the following way:

My house: Do you see my house? It looks beautiful now, but it hasn't always been like this. There was a time when you couldn't enter the house because of all the mess inside. Not that you could see it. But the front door was almost always locked, and it couldn't be opened however much you tried. It's very different now. Flexible and fluent, well greased and oiled, the door opens for anyone who wants to get in. And that's quite something already! If I let people in, I want them to leave their own mess at home or at least to take it back home again when they're leaving. I'm not a charity organization, am I? It's already hard enough to take care of my own clutter and I don't need anyone else's junk, do I? I also like them to wipe their feet. You'd be amazed what they sometimes take inside under the soles of their shoes. You shouldn't expect them to notice it themselves, because they're really blind in this respect. The other day, there was someone who... etc.

The living room: have you seen the living room yet? So beautiful... It's become gorgeous. I've whitened the walls, bought some new curtains, a nice carpet... Have you seen the lamps? There was a time that I didn't even have lamps, or they were broken, I don't know. But take a look at them now... Beautiful, aren't they? Do you remember last year, around this season...? It was absolutely dreadful, don't you agree? It was really necessary that my room be taken care of. I didn't do it on my own. I really couldn't. You think you can do everything alone, and you want to. It's all to do with shame, you know. But I'm glad I got some help. You have to do the main part on your own, that's only reasonable. But that help... I was really glad I received it. I had decorated my living room in a warm and cozy style, it isn't such a mess anymore. I know where everything is as well. Yes, that used to be different. And now I have to keep it tidy and that is not always easy. But I have made a plan, so I really can't escape it. Nowadays, when I see clutter lying around, I ask myself where it's coming from. Sometimes it startles me, because I've brought it with me without being aware of it. It's hard to believe that is possible, isn't it? The other day I saw something lying in the closet, and I had no idea where it was coming from, who had given it to me or whether I had bought it myself. And when. And why. On what occasion and with what intention. I didn't even like it and when I looked at it more closely, it even struck me as very ugly, so how on earth...

The bathroom: It's wonderful. Streaming hot and cold water, very nice. Do you realize how great it is? There was a time when nothing was coming out of the faucet. It had run completely dry. Would you like to know why? When it was finally open, it couldn't be stopped anymore. There was no way I could close it again, an inundation... Terrible! And afterwards it kept on dripping. I guess the tubes really needed a good flushing.
Let's say that all the old remnants from the past had to go. There had been plenty of bacteria that had really thrived and were washed away now, I believe. And then the toilet... One big constipation. After I found out what had caused it – because you do need to know – I flushed out and disinfected the whole thing. It really took much effort to properly disinfect it. For an entire month, I was pouring bleach into the toilet pot. That ought to be enough,

right? Everything is going smoothly now and I would like to keep it that way. But the walls, have you seen the walls? There used to be a crooked wall, do you remember? And a big hole, or rather three holes, have you never seen them? Ever? How is that possible? To be honest, I only noticed these things after some time. It was only after I had bought my new glasses, that I saw it.

The cellar/attic: The cellar and the attic are often dusty, dark, full of strange stuff that you're keeping for some future moment when you are going to need it again. Often outdated, old-fashioned, and sometimes smelly things, discolored, full of holes, not to mention the dust and vermin on it yuck. But you still hang onto it, don't you? What idiot would do such a thing? When I decided to take a look in the cellar to find out what I had been keeping for years, I was really startled. To think that I had been keeping all that! Unbelievable! And sometimes I had really tied it together. I'm feeling embarrassed when I think of it. And the boxes, cans, and bottles, I found so many... I really couldn't believe it. Some of them even were sealed! Like they contained a big secret or something! Well, I guess they did. As if no one else would be keeping cans in his cellar. As if any other person would know exactly what he is keeping in his cellar and why, and if it is supposed to be there. I can still get angry if I think of it...
After the cellar, it was time for the attic, another room you'd better not visit. Crates, cupboards, drawers you could hardly open. I learned it is impossible to throw everything away all at once. I first just needed to live through everything, look at it, sometimes even feel it and smell it, I really did! And only after that was I able to let go of it. Finally! And it is a wonderful feeling, it's really great! I'm still enjoying the relief. I never want to collect such a mess in the attic again. Which led to several resolutions...

Hearing voices
Regarding my hearing voices, psychological processing was filled in a bit differently, but it is possible to recognize the structure of my psyche in the voices I was hearing as well.

I'm hearing something. Is it mine? No, where is it coming from? What does it want from me? What should I do with it? Should I do something with it? Go away! Go away, damn it! What am I hearing? Something bumping? Where is it coming from? Am I going insane? No, I'm not crazy. What is it? For heaven's sake, what is it? Who is calling? Who is saying that? Am I hearing a bell? The doorbell? There's nobody there. Am I going mad? Who's calling? Who's talking, are they talking to me? What do you want from me? Please stop it, you're frightening me. Leave me alone.., please, leave me alone. What do you want? Are you still there? Shall I listen to you? But I'm afraid. What is mine? Are you kind or are you evil? You're dealing with me! Where am I, who am I? What am I hearing? A soft, sweet voice? The voice can hardly make itself heard through all the noise of the other noisy voices. What a noise, what a racket, they're all saying bad things. I'm no good, I'm stupid and very ugly. What is the soft voice saying? 'It isn't true, I'm coming to help you.' Could that really be the truth? Could there be someone who would be making the effort to help me... Oh, if only it could be true. 'I will help you,' the soft voice is saying. I can hardly hear this voice, but I want to hear her. Because this voice is helping me, she's told me so. I'll chase all the scum away and it won't be easy. But the good voice is telling me how to do it. The voice is instructing me and giving me advice.

After I'd made an inventory of my house and thoroughly cleaned it up, the following process was being started.

Writing books
During the phase of organization, I was writing entire manuscripts, my largest manuscript consisting of 360 pages. A tremendous achievement for someone who had never written anything before, and who had lacked any ambition in this respect and hardly knew to express herself in grammatically correct Dutch. I had the feeling I would save the world from destruction (just like many other people who are being inspired, but also lost their way). I would be the one who was going to tell people what was missing in their lives. People did not know themselves, they didn't possess the right level of awareness. For this reason, people couldn't consciously attune to a deeper, cosmic world. Of course, this deeper cosmic connection exists in every human being, just as every human being has the potential of becoming a murderer or a loving personality. Human nature encompasses both good and

bad, human beings possess all possibilities. But in my view, mankind was deaf and blind. I was going to tell mankind how to become more aware. And that was my blind spot, my trap, my ego, if you like, that was not taking into account the stages of consciousness individual human beings have reached. After all, it is impossible to skip a year at school when you're living through the process of consciousness, of wanting to expand one's consciousness, but at the time I did not realize this.

My attack, although in those days I wouldn't have called it that, mainly concentrated on child and youth care. This wasn't very surprising, because the care they were offering my expelled son, whose situation caused me such a lot of pain, was far from perfect. I wrote 360 pages, in which mankind could go on a journey of exploration; it could be compared to a handbook through which people could get to know themselves by means of introspection. To be honest, how could I know they had already written thousands of books and there were just as many courses and workshops about these topics? I sent my manuscript to a well-known publisher (where on earth did I get the courage to do so?) who sent it back to me, commenting that everything was known already. I decided not to be discouraged by this rejection and replied that my book *Social and Psychological Assistance : A Necessary Good or a Necessary Evil* could not be known already. If it were, how could so many professionals fail to cooperate with each other? Why were all of them thinking that they knew better than everybody else? Shortly after that, I received a polite note saying that those professionals generally do not read this kind of book. I somehow found this a good, acceptable answer.

If you think that was the end of my writing career, you're wrong. I wrote another five or six manuscripts, all of which were meant as wake-up calls for mankind. Of course, all of them were soon sent back to me. I really had quite a blind spot, so that I didn't see I really wanted to force people to read 'my books', whether they liked it or not. When I accepted that I couldn't share my knowledge with anyone, and that more than anything else I couldn't change care organizations, I felt an enormous inner peace. Okay, so it wasn't my problem anymore. People had to change themselves, or in other words: they had to realize they had the potential of reaching their true core, their real being. This meant letting go (accepting that it didn't work that way), throwing away (transforming negative feelings and emotions) anything that would impair my personal growth, and embracing, letting in anything that could help me develop my consciousness. It wasn't negative at all; I'd learned a lot from it. For the time being, it simply wasn't meant to be that I'd write a book. Looking back at it, I realize I was not ready yet.

3. With whom do I want to collaborate?

During the phase of organization, I learned with what voices (or layers of feeling) I did or did not want to collaborate. Through the process of writing, of writing it away, of sharing my knowledge, I learned that I couldn't walk a straight path. Only falling down and standing up again, would I discover the right way, would I learn to grow. The so-called 'negative voice' that had led me astray – as no book based on my first writings was going to be published at the time – turned out to have a positive outcome after all. I had to come down and off my pedestal, I had to learn to surrender, to feel trust. My stamina was increased, my will power was redirected and in a similar way, thousands of other aspects of my consciousness were repeatedly analyzed, so that I got to know myself and my way of thinking better. Of course, I'm the one who decides what voice I want to be dealing with. My choice was and continues to be very important.

Many mediums, psychics, dowsers, therapists, and other inspired people can be heard to say: 'The voice is saying', or: 'They're saying', 'My intuition, my feeling is telling me'... They do make distinctions but nevertheless it is often unclear what they're talking about.

According to the mainstream psychiatric model, hearing voices is essentially different. Psychiatrists will always talk about voices, sounds, etc. They often will not refer to an underlying feeling represented by the voice. However, if you start from a psychical model, in my view, every voice symbolically represents a person (living or dead) that refers to a conscious layer of awareness.

At the beginning of my development I received names of people who had known each other in a previous life. The beyond was really influencing my mind even though I wasn't looking for it. For example: Marian had been Peter's brother in a distant past and that was the reason why she could get along so well with him in this life. I also received messages of a deceased personality who wanted to send greetings to someone. For example: Mary is greeting Joe and she's telling me that Joe always took such good care of her and their children. Mary had long been ill and Joe had been looking after her with a lot of devotion and love until she passed on. After this phase of seeing, hearing, and feeling, I decided this really was not what I wanted to do. I made it clear to the voice (spirit) that I didn't want to be available for these spiritual messages any longer.

After that I was often inspired to write a poem or a story. During this period, I still received names sometimes. I also told this voice or layer of consciousness that I didn't need to know any names. Every entity (layer of consciousness) could essentially give me many names if we take the concept of reincarnation seriously. I unequivocally refused to receive any more names and I was possibly inspired to do so by my guide or subconscious. It felt better that way.

I or my soul, my deeper consciousness wanted to do something else, but what exactly was it?

The next step was that I wanted to give a course of intuitive development through painting. The voice explained exactly how I should give this course. And it worked tremendously well. I was receiving impressions of feelings, thoughts, and emotions that were confusing and impairing people. Of course, I didn't want to hear or see everybody's blockages so you can imagine I was having a hard time. Should I really tell them what I was receiving? And even if I did so in a gentle way... sometimes a student didn't want to see or know anything and I learned to respect that.

My father's passing

After I had given a course several times, I wanted to expand my services. However, my father became ill and I decided to stop giving the course. This created some space for the next process. Something which appears to be negative, may still give you space to develop and unfold yourself.

I looked after my father in the last period of his life. My father was a true example of transformation just like many other people (including myself) who have been physically or mentally ill. He used to be someone who was generally self-centered, although he had lots of social contacts, but not within his own family; and now he was mentally reborn through his illness (he had a heart attack, long cancer and prostate cancer). He enormously regretted his former self-centered attitude and he did everything he could to make up for his faults toward my mother. That way, my father and mother had grown closer and closer and after the first tumor had been removed, they experienced 15 wonderful years together in which they shared all the good and bad times. I got or took enough time to take care of my father, together with my mother, during the last years of his life. This was a wonderful experience and my mother and I look back on it with gratitude. During the last days of his life here on earth, my father was in touch with the hereafter and he heard beautiful music.

He saw people (spirits) who had passed on a long time ago, and he slowly flowed from this earth to another reality.

Three months after he had passed on, I was shown what stage my father was living through: he was asleep and recovering from his passing.

After a few months I was told that he was 'awake' and conscious of the fact that he'd passed on. He lives on in the hereafter and continues to learn there. Now and then, he sends me greetings by touching me with a sudden memory that arises out of nothing. My mother also regularly dreams about him, which gives her a lot of strength.

Reading and meditating
After this beautiful experience, I studied an enormous number of books dealing with meaning, spirituality, spiritualism, and emotional development. I used to read two sentences and then I meditated about them for half an hour to understand their meaning. The voice explained how I could interpret things. Each time, we went deeper and deeper until we had reached the nothing and the everything. Here's an example of such a dialogue:
Every human being is God, is divine, how should I understand these words? That we are all minute parts of the bigger whole.

Every human being possesses his or her own Wisdom, stubbornness impairs your development. Does this mean that my soul contains everything? Both what is called the lower and the higher; both the good and the bad? And may I conclude from this that I can choose with my own free will what direction I will take, after which I will perhaps search for balance again? How could I interpret this? I continued thinking and I always received a very alert reaction to my thoughts, which led to an endless number of dialogues:

Every human being essentially carries it inside, it's part of his potential of being. You may regard this as divine, as a power and a force of which you're still largely unaware, let alone that you'd know how to use this positively.

And then I thought: And what about stubbornness? Is it my ego, which often only concentrates on earthly matter, on thinking, on acting based on earthly norms and standards? If so, is this wrong?

You shouldn't be talking about being wrong. When you think of it, in essence nothing is wrong and there are no faults. It is all related to development, to being aware and unaware.

What if my son wants an expensive car, does it mean that he lacks awareness?

No, it has nothing to do with that. He could ask himself what it is that makes him want that particular car. What this says about himself. What he expects to achieve with it or to be because of it. It is not wrong to want an expensive car, not at all. It's a phase, a process of consciousness in someone's life, a possibility for growth.

And that is how our dialogues went on, sometimes for hours. I don't mean I was supposed to blindly believe everything, but it can make you think, to try seeing a certain view from a different perspective. They often went deeper as well, when they were talking about crystallized energies as light, as movement, as feeling that spread in a thousand rotations, and transformed, while at the same time it was located in the same layer. For this purpose, I was shown an inner image of a world full of fascinating colors that shone in the firmament and I understood that we are a part of this. After I had heard about this for a while and had tried to understand it in my own way, to communicate about what was coming through, I also distanced myself from it. This was clearly something for science and not for a simple housewife.

4. What do I want to know?

In retrospect, I think that the deeper layers of my mind gave me more information than I wanted to know. For this, I needed the conversation with a conscious part of myself and my spiritual guide (layer of consciousness). I wouldn't be able to tell what and who was responsible for what parts of my experience. I can imagine that they continually make fresh combinations. After all, the more I, as a human being, know, the more my knowledge gets integrated. What is subconscious becomes conscious, and is led back to the subconscious again. The first time you learn how to walk is not easy. Later on, walking becomes automatic, and you don't even think about it anymore. We see the same process when I'm learning something from my inner teacher who could be regarded as a guide or spirit guide. Whatever I get to learn from 'them' is going to be integrated into my consciousness, if all goes well, and may be considered a part of it from then on. You could say it's a higher school year within your career at the school of life, a school of knowing, feeling, and being.

I wanted, or rather a layer of my consciousness wanted to get to know better and learn to recognize my thoughts, feelings, and emotions. I immediately met a dilemma because I asked myself what part, what feeling, thought, and even emotion was fully 100% my own, and what part belonged to someone else. What is mine and what is yours or his or hers if after all we are consciously and subconsciously interconnected?

Learning to 'think roundly'
The voice told me I had to learn to 'think roundly'. In my manuscript of 360 pages, I described this technique, which is not that important if you think of it. Because if you want to get to know your feelings, your emotions, and your thoughts, you end up in the realm of infinity. All the same, I did seriously attempt to get to know and recognize myself. A seemingly infinite number of words, feelings, and thoughts were written down by me. One way or the other, the actual writing down remains a human achievement! But after that, my guide (although from a cosmic perspective nothing is exclusively mine, as everything is interconnected and interdependent) put me to work.

I was flying up from the earthly world of thought into the cosmic worlds, where boundaries fade away, the boundaries we need here on earth to be able to understand life in all its ups and downs.

"Imagine you have a scale from 1 to 100, how would you rate the value of love? There is material love, physical love, mental love, spiritual love, universal love, self-love, selfish love, love with a double agenda, sexual love, etc. What is it that people regard and experience as love? You can divide everything into positive and negative. One person will value one kind of love as something positive, and another person will consider that same kind of love wholly negative. It's important to realize that there are two sides to everything. Essentially, every person sees the distinction and shares the same insights. However, mankind's stage of consciousness represents its thinking and acting." And so on. Getting to the point, let's take the example of sexual love, which in fact cannot be regarded as a pure form of love but is characterized by feelings like lust and satisfaction, a natural ability to preserve the species. I used to view porn as purely negative, but even in this respect I was corrected by the voice. On a scale of 1 to 100 I ranked porn as 100, i.e., as something completely negative. However, I was told that porn can be viewed as partially positive. A few individuals simply need porn to prevent them from raping women. Some individuals need it to relax. It keeps you busy. Yet another person will feel the urge to critically explore the world of porn. Somebody will want to work in social or psychological assistance because he or she will see the need for porn as something based on lack of awareness, anger, sadness, insecurity, fear, a lack of being connected with oneself.

I found out that my thoughts about this were rather narrow-minded and judgmental and that I needed to change my thinking and views. Anything with consciousness has two sides, which are seen as positive and negative by man. For instance, I saw the word *satisfied* as something wholly positive, but I soon found out it is not. Imagine a person who is completely satisfied, so that he thinks he does not need to do anything anymore and just needs to be fully himself. Such a person will soon run into trouble on earth. Such a person is purely self-centered and doesn't realize that this world, with all its ups and downs, also remains his world. Sometimes it is necessary to be a bit or even very dissatisfied in order to be motivated to change certain things, or to think of your fellow human being who is also a part of yourself, of the common world we all belong to.

And that's how I encountered one feeling after another in all their diversity. Jealousy was another type of feeling I really hated and I thought it was a feeling I should never experience. I learned from my spiritual "psychologist" that jealousy differs from one person to another on a scale of 1 to 100 and that it is not always as bad as I thought. Sometimes, I found someone's house very beautiful and I felt a little jealous that I didn't own that house. Still, the feeling didn't prevail because I thought of the mortgage, maintenance, the surroundings and all the other things that you may encounter concerning a new or different house. I learned that a feeling never is a separate element, as it is part of a larger inner world, a whole scale of feelings that are subject to major mood swings, to changes. Love, earthly love, never is 100% pure, but it always consists, to a certain percentage, of fear, sadness, loneliness, aggression, jealousy, and many other feelings. But even such feelings are necessary so that you won't fully evaporate in space and time. After all, we're supposed to keep our feet on the ground. That's why I had to learn to "think roundly" so that I would be better able to think things through from a deeper context.

Accepting and dealing with 'good and bad'
I learned I really was allowed, albeit only for a limited time, to feel angry, sad, lonely, and whatever else I had forbidden myself to feel. I was writing things down like: I'm angry because my children never listen to me. I'm angry because they don't value me enough. I'm mad because I find my children selfish. I'm jealous of their freedom.
After I had written down my frustrations, which felt good, I rebalanced myself again to neutralize my negativism. Which meant things like: I'm glad my son cleaned up his room. I'm glad my son told me he had enjoyed dinner. I'm glad my son has his own opinion. I'm glad my children may enjoy freedom (within certain boundaries, of course). I now realize that behind their behavior, their frustrations and wishes, there are feelings that I haven't been

able to integrate yet. And I know that the same also holds for myself, because sometimes I can't handle the situation either. Accepting and dealing with things is quite a job, from which you can learn a lot.

At a later stage, I learned that when I was in physical, emotional or mental pain, I had to move closer to the pain. Without judging or condemning, I looked at my pain, and accepted it, which made it flow away or dissolve in time. This was truly miraculous and although I sometimes forgot to apply this method, or it didn't always seem to work that well, in many cases the pain dissolved completely. Most of the time, I tried to avoid pain, sadness, and other negative emotions, I denied them for myself, or wanted to appear strong in spite of everything. This caused muscle tension, cramps, temporary loss of speech, or a common cold. One day, I was considerably emotionally touched and a few hours later I had caught a cold. I felt the cold rise in me, so to speak. I clearly didn't deal properly with the emotions that were flooding me. I didn't let go of anything, I needlessly held on to everything, so that I was subconsciously hurting myself even more. The result was an emotional constipation. It was time to take a close look at my emotions again and learn to let them flow away.

The APL-concept
During the phase of organization, my guide taught me the so-called APL-concept, which stands for accepting, processing, and letting go.

Accepting
First, I had to accept everything I was encountering on my path, whatever I was seeing, feeling, hearing, in other words: whatever I was experiencing. I had to accept everything, and I really mean everything, if only for one second. If I didn't accept something as being a temporary reality or possibility, I was creating a wall for myself that prevented me from looking beyond. I was blocking my own development.

Processing
Processing is an inseparable part of consciousness. You have to process what you're feeling, experiencing, hearing, seeing, or smelling. And this may take

just a second but also a whole lifetime. Processing is something you can't skip, because it constitutes an integral part of becoming more aware, experiencing and living through, so that we're able to let go.

Letting go
Letting go completes the trinity of the process of consciousness. With certain feelings, this may again take only a second, but you may struggle your whole life with other feelings. If you can't let go, you're building your own wall that will be blocking your view.

Well, there I was! It wasn't exactly easy. And as if this still wasn't enough, they also told me: "You'll be dealing with this trinity for the rest of your life. Both at a small and at a larger scale. In difficult periods and during the good times."
For a while, this was hard to swallow. Was it pleasant? Not really. It was instructive though. And I obviously forgot it many times but I finally remembered it every time I'd forgotten it. How could I be so stupid, I'd think, I knew it already, didn't I? Hadn't I received the insight? Well, why didn't I learn from it then? "Knowing and acting constitute a unity, they're inseparably connected," they'd tell me in such a situation. And then I would leave, feeling embarrassed about myself (sometimes screaming, growling, and cursing inside), in order to do my homework.

In reality, I had lived through this process many times already. I described this before in the passages about painting, dancing, and of course writing. Accepting, processing, and letting go of what you're living through so that you can go on again. For me personally, it explains yet another dimension of my emotional life. Emotionally, the blows I had experienced from being bullied at school and, at a later stage, during my divorce, certainly hadn't been too devastating. I rather think of things like my children, the APL-concept that I'm living through, because life would not go the way I'd like it to go. When I think of the course of their personal development, I see this as a kind of rebirth for us all.

Mirror

After my divorce I bought a new bedroom and my guide gave me the instruction to buy a big mirror as well. Both literally and metaphorically I had to learn to look in the mirror. I had not really looked in the mirror for years, only briefly to comb my hair, but nothing more. Apparently, I was thinking: Who doesn't want to see anything, isn't bothered by anything either. I came away with a flea in my ear and I had to take a closer look at myself both from the inside (mentally) and from the outside (physically). And with the help of my guide, I learned to do this better each time.

Mirroring yourself is very important once you're dealing with hearing voices. I hardly saw myself from the outside, let alone from the inside. To be honest, I thought I knew myself quite well, but it turned out this was not at all true. The voice made this very clear to me. Thoughts, feelings, and emotions were rolling all over me, and continually imposed themselves on me. My I was trudging behind them somewhere as in a small, unimportant cart. This clearly was not how it was meant to be. My I was allowed to be there and it really had something to say about things. Of course, I ought not to scream too loud but not only was loud screaming on occasion nonproblematic, but sometimes even – temporarily – necessary. And then, after that, you have to let go again to be able to continue your path.

The phase of stabilization
In the book by Romme and Escher, the third phase, the phase of stabilization, is regarded as a phase in which one has learned to deal with the voice(s). In their view, the voices are to be considered mostly as belonging to the person's own personality, because what the voices are saying refers to the same person who is hearing the voices.

Is this text also applicable to me? For somebody who thinks, or even is certain, that he or she is being inspired by the beyond (a layer of consciousness that is more aware, which in my view is connected to my tiny little part)? Yes, I think so. Of course, the voice belonged to my personal inner world of feeling and experience. A voice can only be attuned to the frequency of feeling that is available to it at that particular moment. A guide, entity or cloud of energy can really connect to any person, depending on the kind of feeling you represent or believe to 'be' at that moment. Therefore, in my view, being inspired is not a unique phenomenon. Regarding myself, there isn't anything new you couldn't learn by any other means. A scientist, a discoverer could add something new, starting from his particular discipline; and I think this would be partially based on inspiration derived from the beyond. As a mother and as a personality, I benefited more effectively from the introspection into my functioning and malfunctioning. Ultimately, I'm helped more effectively by this practice, and the same goes for my family. Stabilizing, getting insight into what a particular voice or frequency of feeling is saying in order to get control or understanding, is, in my view, very important. What is the surplus value of the voice? What is actually being said or what is the intention behind what is being said? And the same questions could be posed for seeing, smelling, tasting, and feeling.

Any psychiatrist may tell you that any person could potentially become a murderer. The same goes for the positive potential in man that is given names such as the divine, the Source, the connection to the All-consciousness, and this positive potential could also develop itself on that basis. "Feeling is being alive, and being alive is feeling," I once read in a book by the Dutch medium Jozef Rulof (*Masks and people*). And I've started to meditate on this sentence in my own life quite intensely, and from a completely different angle.
My guide helped me in this process to develop more clarity in my thinking: "Life is feeling, everything is feeling, although we don't accept this. Feeling is light, space, movement, imagination, color, radiation, and so on. A world you could call both conscious and unconscious. A world that is going from the invisible, the unmeasurable, to the materialized world, so that we learn to expand our understanding of life. It's quite narrow-minded to think that reason and feeling have to distance themselves from each other. Both aspects need to form a coherent whole, if you want to develop as a human being on an emotional, psychical and spiritual level. On the other hand, we do make clear distinctions between things, just as we do regarding all things on earth. Thus, we know, for instance, the opposites of good and bad, male and female, death and birth, the beyond and the earth. From a cosmic perspective, all these things are interconnected and we're living in one world."

The unpleasant part about this, was that I used to be and still am a very sensitive human being. Reading lots of New Age books, I had felt confused during the first stage of my hearing voices. I started listening to my feelings even more, whereas I really needed my rational common sense, and not so much my emotionality, to stay in the here-and-now. I got completely lost in my feelings and mindlessly followed my emotions. I said whatever I was thinking and I didn't draw any lines for self-protection. For instance, I was afraid that my son was doing something wrong and got completely trapped in my fear.

Therefore, my feeling was far from balanced, because my fear was dominating me. After I really suffered the consequences from this attitude, I felt that this wasn't the path I was supposed to go. I heard a new lesson, which wasn't pleasant, but at least it was clear. As an emotional personality I clearly needed to learn to listen more to my reason and grant it a much bigger role in my life so that I wouldn't mentally suffer a fatal accident. Books that carry the message: "Listen more to what you're feeling" clearly aim at people who have a predominantly rational personality.

From this perspective, we may say that there never is just one single answer. Every human being has his or her personal development that can be considered unique. Overlaps, recognition, a temporary coming together, all of this is possible. But after that, each person will have to continue his or her own path, even though you may stay connected to each other to a lesser or greater extent. Compare this to a couple who are madly in love and completely focus on each other. After some time, you will have to be able to function and act separately again, if you don't want to lose yourself. We see a similar process involved in hearing voices. During the phase of stabilization, I learned when I was allowed to receive help from the voice, when I was being influenced or inspired, and when I had to function on my own accord.

During the phase of stabilization I was dealing with the following aspects:

1. Learning to listen to my inner teacher.
2. Making sure I didn't lose or neglect myself.
3. When am I being inspired?
4. Degrees of telepathy.

5. What does the voice (as a source of inspiration) do for me?
6. Renewed insights.
7. Psychology and spirituality.

1. Learning to listen to my inner teacher.
Each time, I learned to listen better to my inner teacher, who continually came to help me when I was going through difficult times. Who explained to me (many times) how I could view something, or how I could analyze a certain incident in a particular manner. "Wrong" is not wrong from a cosmic perspective, but it boils down to a learning process that man has to live through to become detached from it. I learned that I was both a pupil and a (potential) teacher, because I was capable of all possible degrees of feeling. Together with the deeper layers of my soul (that are not exclusively attuned to earthly matter), I was able to connect with my guide/my coach/a higher or deeper level of consciousness, and to tune in to a higher form of knowing and being. My guide (a deeper part of the subconscious) would ensure that I got connected to a frequency of a feeling that was more aware and that I processed numerous impressions. I cannot do this on my own with nothing but my human consciousness, purely focused on earthly matter. It would drive me crazy, because I can't process everything. The cosmos is arranged in such a manner that I as a human being need to be eager to learn things before I really can learn something. If I think I can be anything, I'll soon fall down like a brick, and I'll take my self-built pedestal with me in my downfall.

My inner source, beyond (my) fear, anger, sadness, loneliness, insecurity, and numerous other feelings that we usually characterize as destructive, helps me during the process of growing in consciousness. Here I can find everything I need to heal myself, to heal my negative feelings and emotions. My inner source, my teacher in all this, helps me out.

2. Making sure I didn't lose or neglect myself.
When you become suddenly more or less mediumistic, apparently out of nothing, it is very important not to lose yourself. I learned that it was necessary that I wanted to be human if I didn't want to lose myself in time and space. Otherwise, I might have lost my way completely. My love for my

children, my involvement in all of their problems, my earthy common sense, all ensured that I stayed down to earth.

Thoughts like: I'm here, in the now, at this moment, what am I doing, am I not floating away from the immediate reality, do I remain in touch with Mother Earth – these are resources that keep me in the here-and-now.

Ever more people consciously make the decision that they want to learn to listen to their feelings. Their intuition tells them what they're allowed (or perhaps need) to know, and what they're allowed to say about other people. As far as I know, 'the field', or the cosmos is an open channel from which in essence any human being can get information or to which anybody can be connected. In this context, I would like to refer to the title of Wayne Dyer's book *You'll See It When You Believe It*. I've learned that I first need to believe, if only for one second, to be able to accept what you're seeing, hearing, feeling, etc., as a possible (temporary) reality. It is only afterwards that you can decide whether you want to investigate this, to accept it, or to wait for what's happening next, or to throw it away immediately, even though it's possible you're throwing away something valuable. My I is playing an important role in this process, because I need to determine by myself all the things I want to learn about my own inner world of feeling.

3. When am I being inspired?
The first time I realized that there is more to life than we're able to see with the naked eye, which is focused on earthly matter, was in one word overwhelming. I was being overwhelmed by something I had never read about and certainly had never been looking for. I heard *Faith* and *Trust* and for a while it seemed as if I had ended up in a pink cloud of eternal peace and rest. Before this happened, I had regarded the paranormal as something utterly unhealthy and dangerous. I'd never been looking for it until I had a complete mental burn-out. Only then did I 'accidentally' visit a paranormal healer who treated me. Was I really so special that precisely the right people should be crossing my path? Or was it just a natural process during the specific phase of consciousness I was experiencing? After many years, I noticed that from my perspective to be in touch with another world absolutely

does not mean that you need to be unworldly or even special. Each being is already essentially connected to All there is and is attuned to all layers of consciousness and the subconscious. Therefore, at a conscious and subconscious level, you already *are* being inspired, influenced, or triggered. And this may happen in many ways and from all kinds of frequencies of feeling. Physically, mentally, astrally, spiritually, mankind really has thousands of antennae (aura) that are being worked upon. Man's personality decides (often subconsciously) with what he wants to connect at that particular moment. I noticed that there are numerous courses and types of education that aim at charting the psychological level more precisely. Man is creating everything, both consciously and unconsciously, on his own, which means he is also responsible for his thoughts and actions. Which does not mean this always happens in a pure and coherent fashion, at least not from an earthly perspective. Because to what extent is man carried away, to what extent is he flooded by thoughts and feelings that really do not belong to him, but which overwhelm him temporarily? Part of the mental state, one single little weakness, may bring about something which the person had already essentially left behind a long time ago. This means that something has prevented you from fully integrating the matter - those thoughts, feelings, and actions - into your life.

Where this thinking and these actions are coming from, their origin, could still be investigated a lot more deeply. The spiritual level seldom receives enough attention in this respect. People are often aware of the divine element in themselves, but they may forget that there's always a teacher or a field of consciousness that can reach much further and deeper than what we as a human field of consciousness can register or take in and even more than what we can process.

What source of inspiration may I now see as my subconscious (that represents all frequencies of feeling from 'positive to negative' in balance) and what part could I regard and accept as a higher form of knowing and being? Furthermore, I asked myself whether it really mattered. What is mine, what is yours, and what is his or hers or theirs? I learned that I needed to remain connected with myself so that I wouldn't lose myself. From this perspective, your self-centeredness is very important. What do I, what does the deeper part of my being myself really want?

What I learned is that I have to get tuned in, time and again, to purity and integrity. That I may sometimes make a mistake in the process, is something many people probably can relate to. No person is able to be 100% pure for the simple reason that as human beings we wouldn't be able to live and survive here if we were. We are human beings with positive and negative energies. One day, this frequency of feeling will dissolve into a pure substance. In its essence, which is present at a minute level, we find this in man as our divine core, the foundation from which 'all there is' has originated and been produced.

So I'm continuously being inspired both consciously and subconsciously, but from what frequency of feeling or consciousness is this inspiration derived? If I'm being inspired by entities from higher regions, I always notice this, because I'm speaking or writing in an inspired way. Although I do admit that you also need to create the right circumstances for it. By this, I mean there shouldn't be too many negative energies around me that are taking hold of me. Of course, this is also related to the type of consciousness from which I'm functioning at that particular moment and which is dominating my life. Negative energies seem to have more power and force. I still am triggered by them much too often. This is a gigantic learning process for me, at which I still need to work a lot. During the phase of confusion, I thought I was being inspired, but it often turned out to be my own emotions and desires. Perhaps everybody will experience this sometimes, while learning to deal with these powers and forces. Did I make any errors or mistakes because of this? Of course... because I was in the middle of a learning process. Any human being who is learning something will be undergoing a process of development; nobody can escape this.

Essentially, at the level of our deepest being, it's the positive energies that are in charge. And these energies ensure that I can always find my balance again and grow stronger physically, mentally, psychologically, and spiritually all the time. One precondition for this is that I, my small human I, needs to be prepared to listen to a deeper aspect of being. I can consciously open up to inspiration. A field of higher consciousness decides when I will be inspired and for what deeper reasons. If I'm not being inspired, I'll notice that as well. My answers won't be coming as fluently, I'll stammer, I'll be looking for words and answers; I'll be feeling insecure.

I was told: "Someone else can blow it, precisely because of his self-confidence. A lot of self-confidence can be related to an underlying fear, a form of (abuse of) power, arrogance, anger, sadness, and so on. You may find out in quite a simple way whether your intentions are pure. Why doesn't this feel right? A feeling will arise almost automatically. Look at it and ask yourself if the feeling is adequate or whether it leads to another (core) feeling. It may also be the case that your emotional life is being disturbed by somebody else's remarks. Try to analyze it with your pure feeling, sober and free of emotions, and ask yourself if the remark contains some form of truth. Of course, they may also be the result of the other person's frustrations, anger, sadness, and other more or less unconscious feelings. However, you'll find the answer that is important to you at this moment, in yourself, from the depth of the source." And thus continued these lessons. They didn't seem to reach the end. Therefore, a need for an unconditional resilience is connected to the aspect: *Know thyself.*

Why are there moments when I'm not being inspired, although I do feel what is going on? In my view, you can explain this in several ways, depending on what is going on at that particular moment. You can think:

- I'm being overly distracted by earthly affairs.
- The other person present is not taking me seriously.
- The person in question is not ready to be told something about what I'm thinking, feeling or knowing.
- There is something going on that does not concern me.
- This is what the other person wants and he or she will have to deal with it independently.

4. Degrees of telepathy.
Many things have been written about telepathy. The Dutch medium Jozef Rudolf dedicated a book to the topic (*Spiritual Gift*). Lynne McTaggart (*The*

Field) tells about the many layers of the universal consciousness, the Akashic records, and there are many other books that to some extent refer to some kind of telepathy.

In my own case, I experience that I have contact with an inner world of feeling that is more developed than I can presently understand with my human consciousness. I'm so to speak 'plugged in' into another level and receive 'electricity', information, insights, or whatever else my mind needs at that moment. To be honest, I don't care where it comes from, as long as I can receive it whenever I need it. And it always happens like that. That I cannot or do not always hear it (out of anger, fear, jealousy, fear of pain, and many other 'negative' feelings), is another story. Knowing what I'm receiving, has a psychosocial background. It's purely meant for myself, but of course it also contains a deeper aspect of wanting to become and be a conscious human being. It never is 100% pure because my personal inner world of feeling is always involved to some extent. Would this also count as 'telepathy'? I have no idea. In any case it is not telepathy in the usual sense. I prefer to call it: 'a frequency to which I'm tuned in'.

5. What does the voice (as a source of inspiration) do for me?

To put it very simply, 'the voice' is ensuring that I can go on with my life. The voice has become a source of inspiration.

These insights ensure that my emotions won't overwhelm me as often anymore as they used to do. I've become more aware of my moments of happiness and value them more. It means I have learned to deal with the difficulties I find on my path. That I can see the learning process where I used to see only anger, sadness, impotence, and insecurity. When I first started hearing voices they literally told me: "With joy I'll undergo this process." To be honest, I did find this a little over the top. To me, it was more like a very painful process.

However, I did catch the drift of what was being said to me. I scornfully fulfilled my assignment and I did feel some cynicism while doing so. But... it did help. And that is the most important thing, isn't it? They sometimes say that the end justifies the means, and the assignments or insights I received ensured that I could mentally continue my way. I kept standing upright in my turbulent world with highly sensitive children, who were doing many things that went against the natural aspect of wanting to become and be a conscious human being. Although this process was of course necessary and it still is: because who doesn't know the bad won't know the good either. But it did hurt... Oh, how it hurt me as a mother! Yes, for a while... but then I had to let go. Every human being and of course my children too needed and still need to live through their own individual process of increasing awareness. Thus, the voice led me through different phases to make me aware of my thoughts, my feelings, and my emotions by means of:

- Learning to 'think roundly',
- The APL-concept,
- Making choices,
- Meditation,
- Visualization.

After my inner world of feeling had been completely shaken because I had learned not to judge or condemn, and I had learned the APL-concept, the next step was that I was asked to make a choice. If you don't make a choice, you can't make any progress. They asked me: "What do you want? What do you choose and why? Can you justify your choice for yourself? Why? Please explain. Is it connected to a pure intention or is it impure? Does it serve the universal whole or is it more related to your own little I, surrounded by fear, envy, anger, impotence, sadness, wanting to be something, and so on?" I sometimes get a reprimand from my teacher, but always within a context of love.

We're having discussions for entire days, because I naturally won't swallow everything just like that. They really need to do their best to convince me. I have a clear opinion of my own, although I am open to well-founded insights. Growth, progress, are related to renewed insights, i.e., to change. If you think of it, it is impossible to stand still, because life is movement. However, taking a break to let everything sink in, is also a part of life, if you want to live through everything to subsequently be able to go to the next process. I'm clearly having a discussion with my inner voice, but I wouldn't know to what extent this is being directed by the 'psychologist' from the beyond (contact with the omniscient consciousness).

I experience the world in my own individual way, just like any human being. I accept that what people experience as the beyond is identical to our personal inner world of feeling. You could see it as conscious and unconscious, bad and good for yourself as a human being. We essentially carry all feelings in us, so in principle anything can reach you. I've noticed that I can make a choice regarding what I allow to come through and what I don't want to be dealing with. My psychological state of being, my self-knowledge, my preparedness to learn (when you think you know everything, you really have a problem) are enormously important foundations if I want to be able to 'survive' everything and give it a place in my life. I need to sufficiently understand the information that is coming to me, if I don't want to lose myself. This is clearly a choice that I've made, but maybe this was also programmed into a deeper layer of myself.

The impact of an inner world of feeling that is more conscious has motivated me to expand my vocabulary because this used to be minimal. I really needed a larger vocabulary if I wanted to be able to read and understand more books. Moreover, it helped me in my studies to become a counselor. These studies also served two purposes. On the one hand, I could get rid of my sadness, anger, and impotence through writing, and on the other hand, I was working for the future. Most students found it difficult to describe a suitable case study, while such cases were abundantly available to me.

6. Renewed insights
The voice that addressed me in my inspiration created a totally new inner world of feeling in, through, and with me. From my perspective, they were mine already, but they simply had to be rediscovered. They had to be uncovered or exposed. To be unmasked. I learned to think roundly, so that both the positive and the negative side of my feelings were made recognizable, why they were there and why they were allowed to be there (for the time being). I experienced it as a great breakthrough that I could

90

solve the question of karma (cause and effect). I personally experienced it, of course. If one may consider my son's stigma ADD as negative - as a cause - for himself, for me the effect was a positive surplus value. My love expanded, my stamina, concentration, will power, and so on increased. What looked like something negative turned out to be very positive with regard to my mental development. My second son was quite addicted to soft drugs and again I was tested as a mother to learn to deal with this adequately. Regarding my third son, who was diagnosed with Borderline Personality Disorder, my love only grew even more. Not only toward my son, but also toward many people who are dealing with psychological disorders. I consider a developmental disorder a natural procedure within the process of becoming and wanting to be a conscious human being. No more and no less. Is it easy? No. Is it difficult? Yes. But you learn a lot from it if you're willing to see and accept it that way.

My youngest son, whose life is seemingly going smoothly, naturally developed quite a few blockages as well, because during his childhood all the attention used to go to his problematic brothers. It's just the way it is, I can only do my best. As a family we've learned to understand each other better, our stamina has developed, our insights and love have deepened. Which doesn't mean everything is going smoothly. However, communication is an important part within our family and this way we're trying to find solutions to be better able to deal with our problems. From a cosmic perspective, we're a beautiful family that tries to develop the potential for growth as much as possible. We've learned a lot from each other and we can still learn a lot more. We're all learning and growing, and in my view, this process takes a lifetime.

As soon as one has found the source, the right connection, one can ask for an answer to any question. Once, I was thinking about the fact that we've all had many lives as a man and as a woman, if we accept the theory of reincarnation. Man and woman and male and female are not as far apart as people usually think, and sometimes there is no clear boundary, as we can see with gay people and, in another form, with transvestites and all other transgender variants. When I started to think of masturbation, this line was opened for me as well, because I tried to tune in to it. "Indeed, masturbation amounts to satisfying yourself, the other part of yourself, the male or female part. As a woman you're satisfying your male part or as a man you're satisfying your female part." I actually found it quite amusing that they told me this so explicitly and ultimately found the explanation very natural. Really nothing special, but very normal. Your physical I was looking for unity, just like your emotional I, your psychological I, and your spiritual I.

On another occasion, my attention was focused on the beyond. "If we think of it, the beyond does not really exist," they told me. What do you mean by that?, I thought. "We're living in one world with various layers and states and from this unity, man is constructing the beyond or supernatural life. Meaning that there really is one world that in principle always exists in the now. That you don't know all layers has to do with your consciousness. Your earthly consciousness is limited in such a way that you may understand what you're seeing, hearing, and experiencing. If you're going a bit too far, because your human ego wants you to, it will undermine your psychological well-being. In essence we're living in one world in the now. Past and future do not actually exist, but we need to experience them in order to understand reality. In that sense, we also need to make distinctions, because otherwise life could not be understood by the human mind. If you think of it, reincarnation and being incarnated do not really exist either. After all, as human beings we're connected to all layers of existence and through our interconnectedness we may take on any form that is desirable at a particular moment. But again, this insight and this preoccupation of the soul are necessary to learn to know and to recognize all layers. To be able to make distinctions and thus to see the whole."

Insights of other people
One day, I woke up early in the morning and I received all kinds of insights. These insights were related to a person who was being bothered by negative voices. After quite some time, she still wasn't able to deal with it in a way that would have been effective for her. Because I sympathized with her situation, I received information about it. Of course, this does not mean that everything I'm receiving is going to be true or functional. However, I always find it worthwhile to take a closer look at it, and to see whether I can do something

positive with the information received.

Below there is a summary of a 'reading' I received via inspiration.

Inspiration when I tune in to someone else

It is certainly worthwhile to ask yourself whether these insights might help you get a substantial change in the pattern of hearing voices. Hearing voices is an intense experience that permeates your whole existence. You might say it is time that you were reprogrammed. Your thoughts, feelings and emotions are so overwhelmingly present in your world of existence that they prevent you from functioning normally. And 'normally' means, in this context, to be able to function the way you want to. You've lost your inner peace. Peace can't prevail anymore, because the voices are dominating you.

In other words, you're alienated from your own inner world of feeling. No longer do you love yourself enough. You don't realize that you're a valuable human being. Albeit at a subconscious level, you often let your negative feelings get the best of you, and that is not necessary. Release yourself from it by looking yourself in the eyes, full of true love and trust. Trust yourself. The mistake you're making – and it really is not a mistake, but it consists of a lack of awareness or fear – keeps you from looking at the beautiful properties that you possess. And if you don't see them, I tell you that you do have them. Beyond that anger, sadness, impotence, and insecurity, a beautiful human being is hidden. Look at it, realize this is who you really are, and deal with this aspect of being human constructively.

Inspiration focuses on several people

Every human being has good and bad 'voices' or feelings and thoughts he or she has to deal with. Regardless of whether you locate these inside or outside of yourself, see them as a voice of a person, an entity, a guide, a spirit guide, or as the voice of the subconscious; it touches you, or else you wouldn't be able to connect to it. You might view this as streams of thoughts that continue to run through you: a productive or counterproductive flowing river of thoughts. You might also see it as 'talking' or reasoning. And as talking from your heart, led by your emotional intelligence. This river never stops. However, we often sense how the river gets blocked by obstacles that really don't belong there. In such cases you might see a rock or several rocks lying in the river. The flow stagnates more or less. The river actually always continues to flow, if necessary it will stream over or along the rocks. If we think of our thoughts, feelings and emotions, it's the same pattern as the one we encounter among persons who hear voices. The rocks, the voices, often block a good flow. Somebody who is overly stressed, who's suffering from a burn-out, a person who has too much on his mind, too many problems of any kind, may create twisted thoughts. A pattern may arise from which he or she almost cannot escape. Many people know the phenomenon of "It keeps running in my head." This means you can't find the exit from the vortex of thoughts, emotions and feelings. They continue to play the same CD over and over again, and nothing new arises from it, nothing that would be more meaningful than the old, obsolete songs you know all too well. The person who's hearing voices is confronted by an intense stream of thoughts and feelings that spring from the subconscious. This stream is first translated into conscious feelings and emotions, and after that, they manifest as voices. Whether these voices stem from yourself, from this earthly reality, from the beyond, or from anywhere else really doesn't matter.

Inspiration focuses again on the other person
You sometimes let yourself be overwhelmed by this, sometimes you allow your life to be led by it, while you're forgetting yourself in the process. You forget that you have so much power and strength that you can actually have control over your forces of thought. You can use this river of thought rather than getting flooded by it.

Inspiration focuses on myself
If we return to the river, we have to realize that quite often we first have to get rid of the rocks to ensure a good flow. You've already experienced this when you learned to think roundly and use the APL-concept. To clarify this once more: to think roundly means that you can go not only left or right, but also up and down, and dive deeply or remain at the surface. Think of the shape of a ball. Any human being has to learn to find his or her own way of releasing tension and he or she also has to find a personal method of recharging. You'll have to learn to approach your feelings, so that they will

dissolve almost automatically, bit by bit. Sometimes, it will be easy to remove a rock from the river all by yourself or with the help of another person. Sometimes, the water will continually pound against it, so that the rock ends up showing signs of erosion. And yet on other occasions, the water will be flowing around the rock and it will ultimately find its way back to where it really wanted to go.

Inspiration again focuses (more) upon other people
Every human being has voices. Whether we view these as thoughts or experience them as voices does not really matter. You have to accept this difference if you want to get on, in, and with the river. We all know that we have negative thoughts, but we also have positive thoughts. What do you think about yourself? If you like, make a list of your positive thoughts and then another list of your negative thoughts. After that, you try to make lists of equal length. If you have one hundred negative thoughts, you'll also write down one hundred positive thoughts. If you don't like this idea, you may also limit yourself to five negative thoughts and five positive thoughts. But don't you cheat on me, because you would have more than just five negative thoughts. Your positive thoughts will always be honest enough to tell you so. You may pull yourself into balance by looking at your thoughts, feelings, and emotions without being overwhelmed by them.

Your positive thoughts will help you to chart your negative thoughts, feelings, and emotions. This is often not understood and not interpreted that way. But it is precisely your inner power that activates you to do some introspection. Your thoughts reflect your inner world of feeling at a particular moment in time. This has nothing to do with the beautiful personality you really are. In principle, every person hides behind a mountain of negative feelings. We've hidden our true being under a big load of fear, fear, and ever more fear. This fear is translated into anger, sadness, impotence, loneliness, aggression, jealousy, and so on.

As I said before, each person has positive voices (feelings and thoughts); anyone who says he has not, simply hasn't cleaned up his mess yet. He still hasn't looked at what is being hidden behind all this fear. Your positive voice is pushing so hard against your negative voices that will have to be cleaned up. How you can do this, is something you're going to find out for yourself together with your positive voice.

Below, I'm giving you a few tips so that you can start the process. But in the end, it will be you who is going to decide what methods work best for you. From now on, you're taking charge of your life and you won't be manipulated anymore by your voices, or your feelings and emotions that used to dominate you.

Repeat the following phrases whenever you're going through some difficult times:

- I have a positive voice/positive voices that help me know and recognize myself.
- I'm sure the positive voice is there even if I can't hear it.
- I want to hear the voice, because I know that it's there.
- I listen to the voice, because I know that it's there.

Tips:
- Convince yourself that you have a positive voice.
- Ask the voice to help you.
- Ask for pure insights.
- If necessary, ask for inner peace.
- Ask the voice for advice, and listen carefully to establish if it's really the positive voice.
- Give the negative voice(s) some space to offload but limit this to a certain amount of time.
- Realize over and over again that you have a positive voice that wants to help you.
- Start a dialogue with the voice(s) and demand an explanation of why they are saying something or why they want something from you.
- Any negative remark should be countered by a positive remark. It doesn't matter how small the positive thing is. For instance: "I'm enjoying the blue sky, I'm enjoying a beautiful flower, I've had a delicious dinner, Today I really

did my best, I'm wearing a nice sweater, I've vacuumed the room so that the house is tidy." Show that you can do something and that you are someone. And even when you're lying on your bed, you're doing something positive, because you're thinking. You don't let the negative voices take possession of you. If you risk getting really stressed out, ask the good voice for inner peace. Repeat this as often as you need and you'll be freed from your fear. Believe in that peace, because that peace is also available to you. It belongs to everybody's potential. Allow peace to come into your life and put your trust in it. Peace will make your mind stronger.

Expand these tips with tips from your good voice. You have the power and the force to find yourself back again.

Insight can come to us in all kinds of ways. Films, music, plays, art, your family, your friends, work, nature, and so on. Renewed insights may reach you in a thousand different ways, surprise you, inspire you to view life in a different light. This is the century of personal growth. More and more people will experience it and contribute to the earth's transition to a deeper level of consciousness. Mankind is learning more and more to rely on the personal insights that it is carrying deep inside. This wisdom, a deeper form of knowing and being, is available to every human being. We can reach this feeling, this consciousness, if we leave behind the fear that is still taking hold of us too much. Although in part, this fear is also necessary if we want to keep a balance within our humanity so that we're able to function as well as possible.

When I received these messages through inspiration, I decided that I could e-mail them to the person for whom they could have been intended because I had tuned in to her for a while. Not only were they meant for her, I also digressed to my own emotional life. I told her that I had received insights and that I wanted to share them with her. They can be meant just as easily for her as for me or for anyone else. You can pick some things from it that touch you or that seem helpful to you. Later on, she told me she had felt a lot of support from them. "It seemed as if they were specifically written for me," she told me.

Focusing

In this example of an inspiration you clearly see how my emotional life is being influenced by the now, the past, and a possible future. I focus on someone else but I'm also influenced by my past and led by faith, hope, and love. Now how pure is this inspiration? I think my inspiration is just as pure or impure as that of a physician, an artist, or a musician.

7. Psychology and spirituality

When I got emotionally stuck, I developed physical and psychological problems, and the spiritual aspect in me was activated. I studied an enormous number of books. I began with the books by Louise L. Hay, James Redfield, Wayne Dyer, Deepak Chopra, Jozef Rulof, Neale Donald Walsch, Barbara Marciniak, *A Course in Miracles*, Barbara Ann Brennan, Jane Roberts, Eva Pierrakos, Rudiger Dahlke, Christiane Beerlandt, Ken Wilber, Lynne McTaggart, Ervin Laszlo, and so on. Of course, I was influenced by these books, just as you're influenced by the things you see and hear, and more generally by anything you get in touch with consciously or subconsciously. I wanted to get to know this world of psychology, metaphysics, spiritualism, and spirituality better, and if possible to understand it. Much of what I read really touched me. For instance, a statement by Barbara Ann Brennan in her book about the aura. She states that our perception is always limited to certain frequencies. However, there were also many things that did not resonate with me. They weren't useful to me or I interpreted them in my own way. These studies into the how and why of life have brought me a type of faith that I can build on. It is my faith, and it is not related to any one single existing faith, but it is a mix of all faiths. I picked elements that most appealed to me. For example, Eva Pierrakos stresses in one of her books that we shouldn't be sad and we ought not to be sad, because if we are, we're rebelling against something that exists. Such texts helped me in my process of becoming more aware. Some ingredients might still change in the future. As human beings we are investigators and you taste, know, and recognize as many aspects of reality as possible. A deeper inner feeling ensures that I believe in a better future at which we'll all have to work. But it is also a faith based on the fact that I know and experience that there is a higher, more conscious power, which knows more than what I can understand with my small human reasoning abilities. In my personal opinion, wanting to know, feel, experience, and understand more so that we can put everything in the right context is purely related to the psychical insight of the human mind. The purer you are and the freer you are of human errors (if only temporarily), the purer the information you may receive from the cosmos. In this respect, psychology is closely interwoven with spirituality, the one cannot do without the other. I recognized this idea in many books that analyzed human thought and action.

The funny part about this is that my voice, integrated into my inspiration, used the same model and applied it to my personal identity. Even before I'd read all these books, I had learned about this method in practice. Look at yourself, get to know yourself. I was creatively inspired to engage in a duel with myself.

This completes my short overview of the impact the voices have had on my life. In my case, the main voice was positive and I'm lucky that I was mentally strong enough not to lose my I in the process. If a person is hearing predominantly negative voices, which mostly arise from a traumatic experience, the story becomes dramatically different. Whether there is an external entity involved or not, the way the person in question experiences his or her own inner world of feeling is always essential. If I had been confronted by such traumatic experiences as the ones I have witnessed in other people's lives, I wouldn't have known what to do. But perhaps I wasn't supposed to have been very traumatized and maybe I already lived through such experiences in a previous life.

Other questions

Titus asked me several questions about hearing voices. Most of these have been answered now. Below, I want to answer his remaining questions as clearly as possible and add a few more points.

When was the first time that your voices manifested?
When I think of it, this happened and perhaps it couldn't happen any earlier, after I entered a seemingly hopeless emotional crisis.

How do you explain your voices?

I think that hearing voices is always related to an emotion or feeling. Therefore, I regard hearing voices as something enriching, as an opportunity for insight and growth, although this often isn't experienced that way, neither by care workers, nor by the person involved. Nonetheless, you may consider all voices positive, because they tell you something about what is going on with the person in question. The voice reveals the feelings or thoughts that are blocking someone and may do so via beautiful or ugly imagery and metaphors, and in a disguised or clear and concrete fashion. Whether this leads to a positive change or carries a negative charge, really does not matter in this respect. One way or the other, the voice tells us something, it reveals something of the complexity of the human mind. In case you are hearing negative voices, you would expect that you lack a strong foundation of your ego. But you may witness a similar phenomenon in the case of positive voices, namely when you become overly detached from yourself and your present state of being. Hearing voices always reveals something about the person in question, about the central issues his or her mind is occupied with. What is bothering him or her, what sadness or anger is lying behind the voices, or whatever you possibly accept, see, or hear on another level of existence. Hearing voices may be seen as a psycho-dynamic process that is crying for attention. It does not matter whether you explain it in terms of something physical, mental, astral, spiritual, or universal, because it always tells you something about the way you feel, where you stand in life at that particular moment, what is dominating you (often only subconsciously), what you believe in or value. Whether this is real or unreal, is a different question. Hearing voices may also be considered a form of spiritualism (energy forms), which is being translated into images, thoughts, feelings, and which can be expressed by smell, taste, vision, hearing, and tactile impressions.

According to my interpretation, an entity or field of consciousness may manifest, from the past, the present, and the future. I experienced this myself on several occasions, because I was seeing someone who still hadn't arrived physically. I experienced an entity or inner world of feeling through some kind of energy; some kind of vibration which was so subtle that I really cannot describe it. My interpretation of all this is that my consciousness, for whatever reason, was temporarily expanded so that I saw, smelled, felt, or heard something. For instance: I smelled certain flowers while they really couldn't be seen by the naked eye. When I'm hearing voices, the voices can't be heard by other people either, but they are really present for me in the now.

How do you deal with the voices?
After the phase of confusion, but in fact already during that phase as well, I learned, through the help of the positive voice, how to deal with what I was receiving, seeing, feeling, hearing, experiencing. And this was largely connected to earthly reality, with the problems that I was going through at that moment in my inner world of feelings and emotions. I reached an agreement, a kind of partnership in which we had equal rights. I decide whether I will do something with whatever I'll receive, hear, see, or feel. I decide whether I find it worthwhile, and whether I need or want to do something with it.
If you never listen to someone, he will ultimately stop talking, I thought, and for me, this method really worked, because I could close the door. I tuned in to peace, to silence, to nothing, to an environment wherein I felt good. I visualized a wall (a dome, a round circle or something close to it) which surrounded me and was full of light and love and didn't anything through. Another possibility is that I let anything I hear that doesn't suit me flow out of me. I'd listen to it for a little while (as an observer, behind or in my own created world: screen, cloud, cocoon, and so on) without joining it. In other words, I don't run away from it, but I'm able to let it pass me by. At first, I wanted to know everything, but I noticed that I could not handle it and, of course, also that this is not the purpose of the game called life.

Have your voices ever given you any trouble?
Yes, during the phase of confusion, at the very start, which is about thirteen years ago now. I was too open, too curious, I essentially surrendered myself too much to the voices. The voices so to speak "drilled" themselves into me and wanted to throw my I off its pedestal. In this case you really need a pedestal, you need to be grounded on our planet if you don't wish to be completely snowed under.

"They were the boss, they knew better, they had something to tell me," and my I didn't mean anything. My weak ego was rebuilt again with the help of my good voice, but also because I simultaneously realized that I shouldn't think too highly of myself, because now I was getting help from another form of knowing and being.

Let me clarify:
- Hearing voices started with one positive voice.
- After that, during the phase of confusion, I heard several voices. I can imagine that they were coming from the beyond (frequencies of feeling from the cosmos), because I received all kinds of things I knew nothing about. On the other hand, I can also imagine that there were feelings of fear, confusion, and insecurity involved, so that the whole of what I was receiving was unclear and in fact impure.
- After the phase of confusion, but partially also during this phase, I was dealing with one voice that I interpret as constructive, supportive, and positive.
- I interpret the positive voice as an energy field (guide or entity, if you prefer), but it could just as well have been various guides, each of whom - working from individual disciplines - was focused on the level of development I needed or was allowed to attain.

How come you are able to handle your voices so well and others are not?
My first acquaintance with the phenomenon of hearing voices was above all positive. At first, I interpreted this as a benevolent guide. Also, I immediately located this personality outside myself, and I didn't regard it as something that was coming to me from my subconscious. After I had dealt with an energy form that brought me peace more than once, for me this had become a truth, a certainty, which guided me and supported me while I was learning to handle my problems.
I think the difference between myself and a psychiatric client amounts to the fact that during that period in my life I was sufficiently self-aware so that I didn't lose myself in the process. I did have moments in which I was balancing on the edge, and even took a look at the 'psychiatric kitchen', but I made it all the same. Voices have an impact on my thoughts, on my emotional

life. If people have experienced too much negativism and therefore lose their psychological balance (in some situations you might even call the result a mental paralysis), then, in my view, voices from the subconscious get the chance of breaking in.

Coming from a different level of being, I receive the following message: "This has nothing to do with your true self, but it does in fact reveal how you're feeling, your attitude in life. Fear, anger, sadness, loneliness, shame, an inability to process emotions may lie at the foundation of this."

I was lucky that my personal trauma was related to the love for my child whom I needed to let go. Emotionally and psychologically, I was mostly touched by this.

They're telling me: "Many people who hear voices had a traumatic experience at the physical, emotional and psychological level, which touches them, their personality, much deeper. More intense and deeper are the wounds that they had to experience and those wounds disrupted several levels. That is why such people often suffer from negative voices. But highly sensitive personalities are often depressed as well, or they have a natural ability to hear voices (sounds, vibrations).

"A self-image that is too low, a 'distorted' or unstable way of experiencing reality (the person lives with his or her feeling in two worlds at the same time), make the person in question susceptible to hearing voices, seeing images, etc. This may represent both a positive and a negative value," my voice is telling me. And I have something to think about again.

As I was dealing with a positive voice that helped me in my process of becoming mentally stronger and more stable, I naturally did not want to lose it. Also, I really needed this voice mentally to remain standing. The strange 'coincidence' was that from this period on I had to deal with even more setbacks. However, because of the help I received from 'the voice' I was able to handle this each time it happened. From a cosmic perspective, I regard this as expansion, a learning process, or a growth of consciousness. Apparently I, or my mind, was ready for this 'quick' go-around to a deeper level of consciousness. I see my four children as highly sensitive, which expresses itself in a recurrent imbalance of positive and negative feelings. Crime, drugs, alcohol, self-mutilation, an attempted suicide, are things that you don't take lightly as a mother. And yet I was still standing thanks to the support of a being who was more aware than I.

I got to know a different definition of happiness. Happiness had nothing to do with forcing things. Before all this, if I didn't get what I wanted, I didn't allow myself to be happy. I was sad, disappointed, angry, and at a subconscious level, I was creating those feelings myself. I wasn't aware of my feelings and emotions and I didn't know, didn't accept either, that I carried all possibilities inside. I learned to observe my feelings, to pass through them in order to process them without anger or shame. Only then did I get to know another form of happiness. Because who was I, with my human inner world of feeling, to possess the insight, to be able to decide, what happiness means to me or to anyone else. I was still ruled by fear. Well-meant manipulations from my upbringing, environment, society, faith, and circle of friends, had completely distorted my concept of happiness. Furthermore, I had been born with quite a bit of impatience and rebelliousness. Based on a past life or a preview of my present life, I had no reason to be happy. This meant that as a personality I'd already been doubtful about the existence of happiness and I needed to learn in this life that happiness can be real. I also needed to restore the right balance to find my way back to myself, to my true personality. I already had this in me, but due to too many negative or subconscious feelings I had become alienated from the person I really was and wanted to be at a conscious level. I'd become stuck in the role of a victim, or had become too much of an attacker, or I just wanted to be a negotiator rather than making any choices. It all needed to become more balanced if I wanted to function better. This way, my voice taught me how to deal with myself, but also to handle my voices.

Can you see images of things that others cannot see?
About the same period I first heard Faith and Trust, I was also getting images that couldn't be seen by other people. I interpreted them as images from the past, from a previous life. For instance, I saw a male face with a beard, which disappeared again. I also saw a child standing by a curbstone with a big bicycle. The child wore a little flaming red suit and he had really blond hair. I

saw this child standing outside, while physically I was just looking at a wall. When I walked over to the window and looked outside, I didn't see anything. And yet I had seen this image before my mind's eye. I interpret this as an image from another dimension, because I want to be able to explain it, but other than that it has no use for me. I saw a kind of phantom, a mist, that quickly disappeared from my visual field again. Sometimes it was related to a warning, on other occasions to a memory, a greeting from a deceased person. I found these images very confusing and unclear. I decided I didn't want anything to do with it, as much as possible, of course. I could close this part to a large extent, in the sense that it wouldn't frighten me anymore. I often see flashes of images and look at them, and I feel or consider whether I should do anything with them. I'll wait until things get clearer, and only then will I do something with them if necessary.

Have you ever had any experiences that you would like to call paranormal? What is paranormal? Anything beyond what is visible and audible, which is experienced as reality, is considered paranormal. I don't understand the way internet, telephone lines, or television work either, and there are thousands of other things that I don't understand. I have the same problem with the world of the paranormal. Of course, I do try to understand it, because whether I like it or not, it is part of my life. Hearing voices and seeing images have become part of me, and I want to learn to handle this. Do I see this as paranormal experiences? I don't know. What I do know, is that I'm being inspired and this will also be familiar to many people. Think of an artist or a scientist who suddenly gets to the see "the light." I receive impressions of what is going on, but I decide for myself what I need or rather what I want to do with them. I had to learn to decide whether I wanted to share my information or not. At first, I absolutely loved everything that I was receiving, and the fact that I listened to myself and it didn't feel as if I were saying anything myself. More than once, I was amazed how 'smart' I was. Afterwards, I realized that I did not want this. I didn't want to 'scan' people consciously or subconsciously without being asked. After all, it was none of my concern. Any person needs to live through his or her own process. I probably received this insight from my soul as well. In this very concise way, I learned what was possible, but I wasn't supposed to continue on this path. Suppose you assume that there are many entities or, if you prefer, frequencies of feeling floating around: waves and particles of emotions, and that all of them can have an impact on you. All of this can reach you because you're an open channel. You'd go completely mad, don't you think? And suppose you're seeing or receiving something, how important is that to you? And is it really that important for the spirit, the entity, or whatever you'd call it? Where does this leave me in that story?

I believe that every human being essentially possesses the paranormal potential 'latently laterally' (terms I received from my voices, which mean invisibly sideways). Some need this potential to see spirits to believe in them or be inspired to new ways of thinking. In that case, a spirit or angel manifests in a certain form that is adapted to the needs and beliefs of the person in question. That isn't wrong; nothing really is. I think that all this is necessary to elevate the person to a higher stage of knowing, feeling, and being. I believe that the resourcefulness of the beyond is infinite. I don't want to hide behind a spirit that would be saying something, thereby adding some weight to my message. By now, I have so much confidence in myself that I don't need this anymore. But I do realize that as a tiny human being, I continue to be to some extent inspired by the beyond, because otherwise I would hardly achieve anything. At the same time, they need me, so this increases my value somewhat again. Is this paranormal? I'd rather say that it is a field which is still much too unknown to science. Unknown and often unrecognized, which explains why they hardly make any progress in analyzing this field to understand it better.

Who or what is a medium?
People who are dealing with the paranormal often see themselves as mediums. Meaning that they would be very special and have a gift that is only meant for themselves. On one hand, they are right, in that they can receive things, but on the other hand, you may also analyze the word 'medium' differently. Essentially, a medium is 'just' a channel that mediates or conducts information, like a newspaper, television, and the internet. The way you experience or look at your paranormal power or mediumship is based on your frame of reference. And just as you like one newspaper better than another, mediumship is different for every human being.

It's my conviction that every human being really possesses mediumistic abilities. You'll get more and more access to deeper layers, and you'll learn to sense them and develop accordingly. If you really put some effort into your learning proces and have laid the foundation for it, this will allow you to develop skills with which you can study your subject matter even deeper and expand it. It is the same for your inner world of feeling and experience. About twelve years ago, I got a beautiful example of this. The Dutch medium Jomanda was extremely popular in those days, and she was giving numerous healings in Tiel. Because I had got stuck in more regular circles, I decided to visit Jomanda as well. She has meant a lot to me because she accepted that there is more between heaven and earth and she's willing to express this in the presence of the whole world. At the same time, I noticed that I could also get what I was receiving from her (energy that enabled me to go on with my life) while I was being outside in nature, or even in my own home. In my view it's connected to a way of believing or opening up.

I also believe that any human being can be both good and bad.

In those days, Jomanda used to organize special days on which she invited a group of people who needed her help (you could register for it). I decided I wanted to experience such a day. It wasn't that I was still having many problems, or so I thought, but I simply was curious and decided to give myself a treat. You were supposed to take a present with you, to be given, during the meeting, to a particular person who really needed it at that moment in time. The person who'd receive the present was supposed to pay a personal visit to the person who had given it away. This was supposed to have some meaning for the other person.

I bought a beautiful postcard, which was like a booklet with pictures and poems. It read: *Lots of luck*. During the meeting it occurred that I had to come forward. First, I received a long story that didn't resonate with me. Finally, I was told that I was a very strong personality. I'd been going through quite a difficult process and the worst part was already behind me.

When Jomanda was ready with her story, she gave me a present. To my surprise, she gave me my very own present and I must say I really liked it, because it was a very beautiful card which mentioned and discussed the many aspects of happiness through photographs and poems. In a way, I got my own 'happiness' back and it felt good. According to my own interpretation, it told me that I really needed only myself. I had to seek happiness in myself, in my development, in my inner world of feeling. You are the one who interprets your happiness, aren't you? No one else can do that for you. After a while I decided to give my present to somebody else at my table who was going through some very hard times and who in my view needed the message a lot more than I did. You have to share your happiness, I think, because that's what really makes you happy.

Another incident I got involved in was as follows. I'd bought a booklet by Jomanda and I'd taken it with me. By the end of the afternoon, I walked toward her, as I wanted her to write something in the book. At one point, she was telling us about a new booklet she was writing. I more or less interrupted her and said in a very spontaneous manner that it might have something to do with old Dutch sayings and proverbs that carry a lot of meaning. Then, Jomanda reacted by turning around and saying nothing. To my surprise, some time later, she did indeed publish a book that contained sayings and proverbs.

My interpretation of this incident is that I had telepathically tuned in to her and that I could therefore see or feel what she was up to. I functioned at the same frequency. Is this paranormal? Is telepathy - seeing or feelings things – paranormal? I don't know. It just felt like I was tuned in to her frequency for a while, although I had no intention of doing so, nor did I make any effort to read her mind.

I view Jomanda as a medium who convinced me of the beyond or a higher power, because she was openly talking about it and really believed in it. Some years later, I became more aware of the way she was dealing with the press and television and I didn't particularly like it. However, it was through her that I got acquainted with both aspects of mediumship and I regard this as an enrichment of my insights into the paranormal aspects of being human. I don't consider myself paranormal, but I certainly am in touch with the paranormal.

Have you ever had any experiences you might call psychotic?
Yes, I had one experience of that type. As I was living on welfare, they obliged me to start looking for a job. At that moment, I absolutely could not handle this, because my situation at home was still very complex. When I told them I was having many problems with my children and was living through some really hard times, they belittled this and termed it 'irrelevant' to my present situation. Time and again they intimidated me, stating that my attitude would have serious consequences for my income and that I simply would have no choice but to start looking for a job. Under these circumstances, I started suffering from anxiety and delusions, which I experienced as very psychotic.

One day I was sitting in my car, waiting for my son, when I was overwhelmed by an immense fear. In the distance, I heard an airplane and I thought it was going to crash down on me and pierce through me. I blenched, taken by fear, as I 'saw' a plane and had the delusional experience that it was furiously crossing over my car, making a tremendous amount of noise. However, the recurrent sound turned out to be the loading of a truck.
Next, I saw a man in the distance, who was approaching me and I was certain that he was going to drag me out of my car. I locked the car door and took on a fetal position to protect myself; to be a child again. The man simply walked on.
There were also other men whom I suspected of coming after me. I suspiciously followed their movements. And nothing happened.

This strange incident took place when I no longer felt safe in the world I was living in. They forced me to do something against which I felt an enormous inner resistance and they did not take this into account. I simply was not heard as a human being, I wasn't taken seriously, I wasn't valued or respected.

When I had this experience, I 'flew away' into various inner worlds of feeling, so to speak. The experience as such lasted about twenty minutes. I was extremely frightened, but in between my fears I was able to observe my own behavior. The illusory images and feelings alternated with reality.

When I look back at it, I can say that this experience was positive, for more than one reason. First of all, my welfare consultant started seeing me more as a human being and taking me more into account. Apart from this, I see this experience as an enrichment of my experiential expertise. Although this short experience certainly cannot be compared with the state of mind of someone who systematically suffers from psychotic experiences, it did give me an impression of how it must feel. A delusional world that to the person who is undergoing the delusion seems real, and which is caused by problems he or she can't handle. I interpreted this incident as an experience I was allowed and needed to have and during which I was being coached by my guide so that I wouldn't sink too deeply into this inner world of feeling.

Looking back at my mental development, the phase of confusion would certainly qualify for the label "psychotic." I don't mean to say that one cannot overcome this state or integrate it into a deeper aspect of being. This is how I think about it and of course I'm being inspired again: If you start from the idea that the human mind contains for instance hundreds of layers and that all human feelings possess hundreds of nuances, you know that there is a limit, that leans over toward the negative. This limit is often misunderstood by the environment, but the person him- or herself can't really grasp it either. The person in question is being overwhelmed by feelings and emotions (images, sounds, etc.) and cannot identify these, which may cause various responses. A human being who is functioning less than half as a human being, becomes some kind of animal and defends his territory. He wants to exert power over other people by acting out his drives, assertiveness, wish to take possession of things, the victory of the species. It is a natural process which has a certain value, but if it rules the human being in question, there is a problem. If this development goes on, you reach a form of consciousness that one could characterize as the plant level of consciousness. If we imagine a tree, we realize that it can only stretch out its roots onto a particular layer of the soil, in which it is anchored, and that's the only way it can assert itself. If a human being is stuck in a specific layer of consciousness or if he doesn't want to reach any further, he'll perish in the world that he created himself and wants to maintain (often subconsciously). The safe haven becomes a prison of the person's own mind. If you look at it, human behavior, not being allowed or not wanting to do anything, wanting to be something or launching an attack, are all connected to the psychological state of the person in question. As human beings, we're all dealing with feelings that we haven't lived through yet, so that we don't have a hold on them yet and haven't learned to handle them yet.

That's all there is to it and it should be treated and approached from this perspective without putting a label on it. If you start from the idea that mankind is developing, within an enormous growing process without equal to get to know itself better, this doesn't agree with the way regular care workers usually view human beings. If it did, I would have had no difficulty in asking for help during my process of confusion. As it was, I didn't even dare take the risk. If you think of it, I was just going through a process of development and integration. No more and no less. I wasn't ill, but I did need help. Just like any other human being, I may be overwhelmed by anger, sadness, impotence, insecurity, confusion. Looking at all this from a cosmic perspective that reaches further than earthly views, which still are overly anchored in societal thinking and acting, I'm able to re-balance myself.

Are you affiliated to any society or foundation that deals with hearing voices?
Some years ago I became a volunteer of Foundation Resonance (Stichting Weerklank).
This foundation is the Dutch organization that struggles for the interests of people who hear voices. Resonance was established during the first congress ever for people who hear voices, held in Utrecht in 1987. Research has shown that 2 to 4 % of the population hears voices. Resonance states that hearing voices is normal, but that you may develop psychological problems if you don't keep them under control.

Resonance is a foundation that aims at all aspects of hearing voices: mental, psychological, emotional, and spiritual aspects, so it really is the place to be for me.
To my surprise, I noticed that most members of Resonance have a psychiatric background and have lived through several admissions to a psychiatric

hospital. However, I also noticed that we have a lot in common, such as hearing voices, seeing images, feelings, and so on. The thing is, with most of the members of Resonance, the negative voices seem to be in control and then it will be an altogether different story.

As a contact person of the aid phone service I was regularly contacted by people who got lost in spiritualism and spirituality. They often have a mediumistic gift, but they don't understand their gift adequately. These people are often misunderstood by regular care institutes. The person who hears voices puts himself on a pedestal, or he hands over his life's scenario to a higher spirit, entity, or for instance, to a spiritual leader he knows from the Bible or other scriptures. They overly identify with the entities that are coming through and can't make a distinction anymore between themselves and others. Crisis management needs more insight into what might be going on with these people and what is possible in this area. By the way, I don't mean to say that any person can be helped. However, to a large extent, it is possible. More insight into what is going on and what the client's needs are during this phase of his life, such as the attunement of the person in question, his views, and several other relevant factors, is really necessary so that the client can deal with the problems at hand. Time and money often play much too big a role in care and this can have disastrous consequences. Growing stronger spiritually and learning to look with insight at everything that's going on, takes time, often lots of time. Consciously and subconsciously, you attract all kinds of things and seen from a spiritualist perspective this can reach very deep and far. We really need an adequate mental health care and there is a real wasteland here for any care-worker to develop.

My love for my fellow human being motivated me to become a member of Foundation Resonance. "Hearing voices is not a disease, but it can make you ill!" is the statement that appeals to me the most. I personally want to stress the aspect of the positive, mind-expanding, insightful voice. In my view, this is only possible if you get to know and recognize yourself better and you reject your low self-image so that you can be reborn.

I have been part of the board of directors of Resonance for some time. I can be reached by phone or e-mail for people who need help or information. I'm also trying to find out if we can start more self-help groups for people who hear voices and possibly for their relatives as well. After all, you can learn to handle your voices if you get more control over your personal inner world of feeling and understand it better.

In my view, good mental health care that aims at hearing voices, but also seeing images, smelling, tasting, and feeling that another person can't perceive, is hard to achieve. They still use the disease model on too many occasions, and the client is not allowed to talk about hearing voices. Approaching what is going on from a very one-sided perspective, they'll soon prescribe medication and they rarely use cognitive therapy and related methods. But even then, the content or meaning of the voices is often not explored during treatment. Medication may certainly have a positive value, but the negative aspect, that of substance dependence, will obviously never lead to a healing of the person in question.

Many ways of becoming or being whole are suitable to help people who hear voices. I personally experienced that I could not avoid the confrontation with my inner world of feeling and experience. Through creative therapy led by my inner teacher, meditation, visualization, learning to think roundly, the APL-concept, confrontation, introspection, reflection, silence, dialogue, monologue, I've learned to recover.

If a care worker gets to know and recognize himself better (which is often part of his education), finds true inspiration, feels and hears from the inside, he or she will ask for methods that are best suited for this particular client at this specific moment in time. After all, from my perspective, he or she is connected to the source of deeper feeling and this doesn't need the label of spirituality. The amount of love, the universal love for yourself and your fellow human being, is in fact the most important part. Because we will be confronted by all kinds of obstacles on many occasions in our lives – after all, this is our learning process – there remains a lot to be learned. And that's what makes life exciting (I wouldn't use the word pleasant) and a challenge to be met.

Foundation Resonance, the books by Marius Romme, Sandra Escher, Ron

Coleman (also see the list of references in the first part of this book), who have earned their reputation in the field, break through this circle and show you a different view on the phenomenon of hearing voices. I'd also like to demystify the word 'phenomenon' by stating that hearing voices (and feeling, and inspiration) can be a natural part of the process of wanting to become a conscious human being. Even if the voices are experienced as negative, they create a potential for insight, and for developing your personal inner world of feeling and experience. For many people, this is and remains a difficult process, wherein a care worker can play a significant supportive role. A care worker should regard the voices as a source of knowledge rather than reject them as a non-existent delusional reality of the person hearing the voices.

What is your present stance on hearing voices?
For me, hearing voices has in fact long stopped being 'hearing voices'. I see it as an interaction with the universal source of all of us. I'm the one who receives messages from the cosmos, and I will ultimately decide for myself what to do with them. Do I see this as a guide, as an entity? To be honest, I'd rather view it as an energy flow with which I'm connected by nature. At this specific moment, in this phase of my life, I have a connection and that's what I need now. You may regard this as a guide who mostly coaches me during a psychological process that incidentally touches upon the spiritual world as well.

I regard spirits, a spirit guide, a helper, as a resource, a metaphoric image if you like, to help mankind on its way to a deeper consciousness. To establish contact to the divine element in ourselves, the subconscious.

My voice stopped being a voice a long time ago. The voice, which is nowadays my source of inspiration, taught me to change my views of the world so that I could better handle my problems. It should be clear by now that the messages from the voice aim at my unique personality. In that sense, I believe that any human being may be helped in his own unique way by balancing his thought and feeling. It is not a coincidence that emotional intelligence is receiving an increasing interest during the last few years. If we want to be able to make the right decisions, we cannot and should not switch off our feelings.

Why exactly did you receive your voices at that particular moment in time?
It is of course related to an emotional, psychological blockage, but also to a
spiritual expansion. As I was, at the beginning of my development, hearing a
voice outside and inside myself, I was confronted by past lives, I was seeing
many things pass by or was being touched by them, I knew that 'the voice'
was necessary in a particular phase of my life to convince me that there is
more between heaven and earth. In principle, every human being is dealing
with a voice, or what is usually termed one's own thoughts. From these
thoughts, your cognitive framework, you're being inspired at a conscious or
subconscious level. For me, hearing voices is related to the biggest antithesis
in our experience: that between *love* and *fear*. If one is being animated out of
love, we often call this inspiration. However, inspiration can also come from
the subconscious or the negative side and it embraces countless degrees. It
may even derive from two sides simultaneously, which raises the question
what the main goal was at that moment in time.
For instance: a man is being inspired to start a certain project that will bring
loads of good things to mankind. This turns out to be an enormous success.
However, at the same time, his family is suffering because he puts his family
second. Things are escalating at home, and there are many problems.
Therefore, inspiration may have many different backgrounds and is connected
to a person's frame of consciousness. Whether the person himself and his
environment see this inspiration as something positive or negative, depends
on the frame of reference from which each person reacts. Hearing voices, or
inspiration, can in most cases be experienced as something enriching, as an
awareness in which you can discover a lot. However, a human being does not
by definition need to see or hear things to be connected to a deeper
consciousness. Love, ranging from universal love and love for yourself to
love for your fellow human being, ensures that you get automatically tuned in
to a deeper aspect of being. Regarding my own voices, I had to deal with
both components. On one hand, the occurrence of voices as a result of
trauma, although I need to stress once more that it all started with a positive
voice. On the other hand, we were growing, as a family, toward a deeper
consciousness and we needed to learn how to deal with this.

In my case, hearing voices, transformed into inspiration, has become something very familiar now. It is nothing special, but it's really quite normal, as soon as you've found the right channel. It's a part of my life, it doesn't dominate me, but it provides insights, and that's all there is to it. And let's be honest, quite often I'm very pleased by my connection. It gives my life more meaning and protects me to a certain extent (there are still processes that I simply have to go through). That's why I persevere in life, why I'm still standing, and that is really quite something amidst this unconscious world growing toward consciousness. And of course I experience plenty of moments and forms of happiness and their number is increasing. Isn't that wonderful?

What's your view on mental health care in this respect?
My own experience with other people who hear voices and ended up in psychiatry is that all too often, the care workers use a lot of medication and the client does not get the chance of talking about his voices. In my view, they should look more at the *reasons why* people hear voices. It is my personal experience that people who end up in psychiatry have usually gone through something traumatic. The trauma often returns as a reflection in their inner world of feeling and experience.

At that particular moment, the client is not able to detach from this inner world of feeling.

Medication is a necessary good and a necessary evil. On the one hand, it is good because it helps us, makes us better, or saves us (keeps us away) from a lot of misery for some time. On the other hand, it is evil because it may (in case of prolonged and thoughtless use) keep us away too long from a process that we will have to struggle through, if we want to make it our own. Medication often blunts or changes our inner world of feelings. Sometimes this is good for a while, but it also leads to many bad things.

Both the client and the care worker will have to be aware of living through a blockage, if they want it to disappear. Of course it depends on the personal situation how deep and how often this should occur. You encounter the same thing among war victims. In times of war, human beings often are strong. A natural motive, survival of the species, manifests itself. However, many develop all kinds of twisted survival strategies. The environment and also the person him- or herself aren't aware how deeply 'walled in' his or her pain, sadness, aggression and so on have become. After the war, these experiences will have to be processed, so that they can be effectively integrated at a deeper level.

Of course, every experience and conflict differs from person to person. If something is traumatic for one person, it does not mean it also has to be traumatic for someone else. This is related to one's state of mind, the subconscious (integrated) insight or the empathic and intuitive power one has. The more spiritual the person in question is, the less he or she will remain stuck in the trauma, and the more he or she will want to let go of the emotion. On the other hand, some people may cling so strongly to the spiritual seeing, acting, and thinking process that they may themselves cause blockages in this respect.

According to several persons who hear voices, present-day mental health care amounts to diagnosing someone based on his or her voices and prescribing medication. The care workers don't explore the voices and the problems they imply. They often don't ask the client anything about possible other problems either.

What I know about alternative approaches to care is that they often remove 'negative' or unconscious energies to re-balance the client's emotional life. Afterwards, the client would have to work on him- or herself, with or without external care, to analyze - via the APL-concept - his or her problems. This type of care often works a lot better with children, because they're still at a different level of consciousness.

Nowadays, we know a lot about spirituality and spiritualism thanks to the countless books that have been published about these topics. Some people seem to think that anyone who has read about these subjects should be able to give a course or workshop just like that, or automatically be capable of constructing an appealing world view and more or less believe in it. In my view, it's important that mental health care workers gather more information about these things. They need to develop more knowledge and become aware of the ins and outs. Psychological insight is strongly interwoven with the development of your spiritual powers. Reading hands or toes, physiognomy, color therapy, aura-readings, iridology, Tarot cards, angel cards, intuitive creative therapy, and so on, all relate to a psychological element in ourselves. If mental health care has more insight into emotions, psychology, spiritualism, and spirituality, one can put the client's questions into the right perspective. It is my impression that alternative and mainstream mental health care are blending into each other more and more. This makes it possible to get the best from both. However, seen from an economic and societal perspective, recognition of the alternative practices will still take quite some time and effort. Both with mainstream and alternative care, it is important to stress that care workers must not use any type of coercive manipulation, because this would impair full integration of knowing and feeling. A large amount of love, combined with a strictness in one's approach, is necessary if one wants to give the right treatment.

What types of (mental health) care are effective nowadays?
Care workers who:
- take enough time to build a relationship based on trust;
- take a client who hears a voice, sees images, experiences or feels something, seriously;
- approach medication as a possible temporary resource, and nothing more than that;
- regard healing and alternative medicine as a possible resource, and nothing more than that;
- use cognitive, communicative, and creative therapy (imagery, visualization, meditation) as methods to reach insights;
- have read quite extensively (even if they are mainstream care workers) about spirituality, spiritualism, regression, and reincarnation, in order to better understand the person who hears voices;
- know their limits and are open to other types of care;
- are not afraid of the emotions evoked by the voices.

In conclusion
Regarding myself, I can say that I've experienced hearing voices as something

enriching. Only since I started hearing voices did I learn to think deeper, and to examine my world view. I learned to silently tune in to the flow that focuses on the universal aspect of being human. Beyond my emotions, I learned how to reach a deeper level of feeling from which I could gain more insights into the how and why in my life. This flow ensures that I won't emotionally crash anymore, which used to be the biggest problem in my life. On the other hand, I do often need my emotions to really make an effort for something, to do my best for it. But I won't get carried away anymore, I won't be overwhelmed by this enormous mental force anymore. Of course, I'm not ready yet, and I even have the feeling that I woke up only recently and that I'm only living consciously since that awakening. I've left kindergarten behind me and have also passed primary school. I'm in secondary school now and it isn't easy. I've learned I need to do my homework every day (tune in to a deeper aspect of being) and if I do, I'll make it. In fact, I won't be so easily upset anymore about anything or anyone as I used to be. I'm the one responsible for my homework. And only then, after I'm ready, will I be allowed to go "play outside" and decide what direction I want to take.

Learning to listen to the voice has become easier every day. This does not mean everything is perfect. But I know how to re-balance myself if things seem to go wrong. When I started a course some time ago that I found very interesting, I felt no motivation whatsoever. It didn't surprise me when after a few months the course was canceled out of the blue, completely unexpectedly. Most students rebelled but it was okay with me. I thought it simply had to be that way. I was given more time and space for other issues that cosmically were much more important for me, at that moment in time.

Essentially, I have the feeling that I have once more been reborn into my life. Since I allow myself to be led by a higher level of consciousness inside, life seems to take its own course. I look at the obstacles and impairments on my path and know how to handle them. Thanks to 'my voice' I've taken an entirely different view on life and experience life in my own unique way, which aims at a deeper level of being human. I have overcome my depressive thoughts and am looking forward with joy and interest to anything life still has in store for me. This doesn't mean I don't have any fears. A healthy dosage of fear is necessary, if you want to rationally analyze what is happening. Take it into the light in order to understand it, process it, and let it go. Otherwise you might become overly confident, and the ego would get involved too much. Someone who's being inspired by the higher, deeper, or more conscious part of the universe, will always have to deal with a healthy amount of fear. This is necessary to re-balance thoughts, feelings, and emotions to be able to continue your path with confidence.

As human beings, we need the rhythm of day and night. The sun (the light, insight) never disappears, it is always present, and at worst, it is hidden behind the clouds (my thoughts, feelings, and emotions). I'm glad I've learned how I can let this light shine again in my life. It was and is always there, it has never really been gone.

About the authors

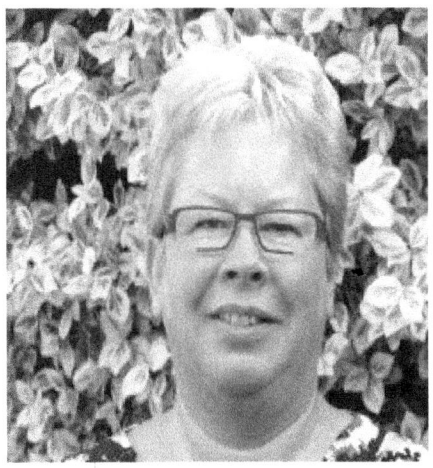

Tilly Gerritsma (1953) is a mother of four sons. She has been a member of the board of directors of Foundation Resonance (Stichting Weerklank) and gives lectures and workshops about hearing voices and extrasensory experiences. See: http://www.stichtingweerklank.nl

Being a mother of four sensitive sons, she is active for a foundation called 'Familie als Bondgenoot' (FB), sharing her experiences as a mother with Dutch mental health care (Geestelijke gezondheidszorg, GGZ) and giving tips about how (not) to deal with it. Together with a colleague, she gives workshops about writing down one's personal experiences. See: http://www.familiealsbondgenoot.nl

Tilly also writes columns about the funny daily things of life, to keep her life in balance.

Tilly Gerritsma can be reached at: megerritsma@online.nl

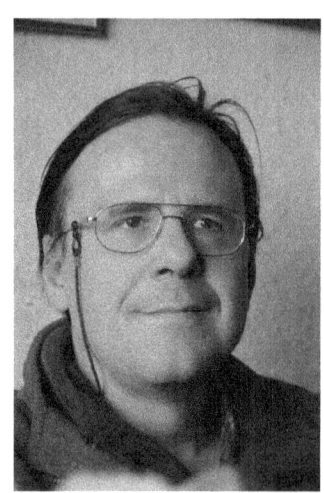

Titus Rivas (1964) is a psychologist and philosopher and works as an author, investigator, and lecturer. He is affiliated to Athanasia Foundation and Merkawah. He has published articles and books about a range of topics from the fields of psychical research and parapsychology, psychology, and philosophy.

Together with Dr. K.S. Rawat he wrote *Reincarnation, the Evidence is Building*. With Anny Dirven he published *Vincent, Karim en Danny*, about paranormally gifted boys, and *Van en naar het Licht*, about Near-Death Experiences and related phenomena. He also co-authored two other books about mental health and care: *Geen goed leven, geen goede dood,* and *Brokkenmakers in de GGz*, both available via Lulu.com.

Titus Rivas can be contacted via: titusrivas@hotmail.com

www.ingramcontent.com/pod-product-compliance
Lightning Source LLC
Chambersburg PA
CBHW081355280526
45788CB00009B/2886